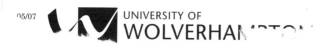

UNIVERSITY OF
WOLVERHAMPTON

Researching ageing and later life

Researching ageing and later life

The practice of social gerontology

Edited by
Anne Jamieson
Christina Victor

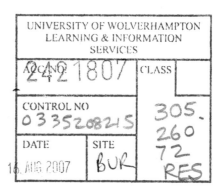

Open University Press
Buckingham • Philadelphia

Open University Press
Celtic Court
22 Ballmoor
Buckingham
MK18 1XW

email: enquiries@openup.co.uk
world wide web: www.openup.co.uk

and
325 Chestnut Street
Philadelphia, PA 19106, USA

First Published 2002

A catalogue record of this book is available from the British Library

ISBN   0 335 20820 7 (pb)   0 335 20821 5 (hb)

Library of Congress Cataloging-in-Publication Data
Researching ageing and later life : the practice of social gerontology / Anne Jamieson and Christina Victor (eds.).
        p. cm.
    Includes bibliographical references and index.
    ISBN 0-335-20821-5 – ISBN 0-335-20820-7 (pbk.)
        1. Gerontology–Methodology.   2. Ageing–Research–Methodology.   3. Old age–Research–Methodology.   I. Jamieson, Anne.   II. Victor, Christina R.
    HQ1061.R452 2002
    305.26′072–dc21

                                                                    2002021405

Typeset by Graphicraft Limited, Hong Kong
Printed in Great Britain by Biddles Limited, Guildford and King's Lynn

Contents

List of figures, tables and boxes

Notes on contributors

The editors

Both the editors are at the University of London and have previously co-edited (with S. Harper) *Critical Approaches to Ageing and Later Life*, Open University Press, 1997.

Anne Jamieson is Senior Lecturer in Gerontology at Birkbeck College, University of London, and course director for the programmes in gerontology, including an MSc in Life Course Development. Has published in the areas of comparative aspects of health and social policies, evaluation studies, and adult education.

Christina Victor is Professor of Social Gerontology at St George's Hospital Medical School, University of London; Dean for Postgraduate Learning and Teaching and course director for two MSc Courses (Health Sciences and Public Health). Has published widely in the social and health aspects of ageing.

Other contributors

Andrew Blaikie is Professor of Historical Sociology, University of Aberdeen. Interests include the social construction of popular images of ageing. Currently researching relationships between culture, biography and memory.

Margaret Boneham is Principal Lecturer in Applied Social Science, Bolton Institute. Previous research on ageing and ethnicity, evaluator of 'Better Government for Older People' project in Bolton, currently working on research into social capital, gender and health.

Joanna Bornat is Senior Lecturer in the School of Health and Social Welfare, The Open University. She is joint editor of *Oral History*, and has researched and published on reminiscence, oral history, ageing and stepfamilies.

Bill Bytheway is Senior Research Fellow in the School of Health and Social Welfare at The Open University. His research interests include issues related to ageism. He is a founder member of the British Society of Gerontology and was editor of *Ageing and Society*, 1997–2001.

Peter Coleman is Professor of Psychogerontology and holds a joint appointment between the Department of Psychology and the Medical School (Geriatric Medicine). His research interests focus on issues of development and adjustment in later life. He was previously editor of *Ageing and Society*.

Jo Cooke is Coordinator for Trent Focus at the University of Sheffield. Among her interests are ways of promoting the use of evidence-based care in the health and social services.

Mary Gilhooly is Professor of Health Studies and Director of the Centre of Gerontology and Health Studies at the University of Paisley. Present research is in the areas of health, quality of life and successful ageing. She is currently President of the British Society of Gerontology.

Mike Hepworth is Reader in Sociology at the University of Aberdeen and Visiting Professor of Sociology at the University of Aberrtay Dundee. He is currently researching images of ageing in nineteenth-century painting.

Julia Johnson is Senior Lecturer in the School of Health and Social Welfare at The Open University. She has been involved in practice, teaching and research in gerontology for the last 25 years and chaired The Open University course, An Ageing Society.

Ann Netten is Director of Personal Social Services Research Unit and Reader in Health and Social Welfare, University of Kent at Canterbury. Research interests include evaluation of health and social care of older people, cost and outcome measurement, informal care, and economic evaluation of criminal justice.

Mike Nolan is Professor of Gerontological Nursing, School of Nursing and Midwifery, University of Sheffield. Interests include the development and evaluation of services for older people, and is currently exploring the dimensions of relationship-centred care.

Sheila Peace is Senior Lecturer in the School of Health and Social Welfare at The Open University. She has written widely in the field of social gerontology, residential care and environment and ageing. She was also the editor of *Researching Social Gerontology* (1990).

Dorothy Sheridan is Head of Special Collections, University of Sussex. She has been Mass-Observation Archivist since 1974. She teaches, researches and publishes in life history, social research methodology and twentieth-century British history.

Michael Wadsworth is Director of the MRC National Survey of Health and Development (the 1946 national birth cohort), visiting professor at the Department of Epidemiology and Public Health, University College London. Research interests include life course studies of health.

Introduction

Anne Jamieson
Christina Victor

Social gerontology is a diverse and heterogeneous academic activity that includes researchers from a broad variety of disciplines. As this book illustrates, not only are the range of questions posed by gerontology extensive, but the range of methods and data sources used to answer them are equally diverse. This book represents the result of collaboration between the editors and the British Society of Gerontology to develop a volume to complement the well-established book on research methods in social gerontology edited by Sheila Peace (1990). In combination these two volumes demonstrate the breadth and diversity of social gerontology in Britain. Our aim, in producing this book, was to update some of the aspects of research where there have been significant changes and to reflect the major methodological innovations that have taken place in the past two decades.

The audience for this book is broad, including researchers and students of gerontology from a variety of different 'home' disciplines and at various stages of development. The chapters are written in a 'practical how-to' style, pointing out the potential of different sources and methodologies. Each chapter provides practical examples of the use of the source/method and reference is made to relevant sources. An appendix lists a wide range of useful websites. As well as being stimulating it is intended that researchers will find this a useful addition to more theoretically focused research methods textbooks.

The book is in four parts. Part I introduces the field of social gerontology, its institutional and theoretical base. The second chapter sets the scene for the reader by discussing the different sources and methods which are reviewed in the remainder of the book. Part II gives examples of the many ways in which researchers make use of existing sources, whether quantitative or qualitative. Part III has examples of different uses of new data collected from individuals, young and old. Part IV addresses the wider issues of the roles of the researcher, both in relation to those being researched, and in relation to different stakeholders.

In developing this new book we have responded to three trends that have characterized British gerontology in the last ten years or so. These are *theoretical* developments, *methodological* developments and changes in the *context* within which research is undertaken. In *theoretical* terms social gerontology has begun to widen its remit, as discussed by Jamieson. The focus initially was upon describing the nature and characteristics of old(er) people. Hence the sources, techniques and methods used were often descriptive in nature, and much research was concerned with establishing the 'problems' of old age. This volume represents the more sophisticated gaze now pursued by gerontologists that looks at later life within a life course context and that is examining the nature of ageing as well as the nature of old age. Life history or biographical approaches continue to be relevant within this context, as illustrated by Bornat, but this volume also includes work on longitudinal birth cohort studies by Wadsworth, and a discussion by Coleman of recent developments in the use of psycho-biographies. His use of the case study approach within a psychological context demonstrates the innovation in theory and method that has taken place over the past two decades. Admittedly, there is still scope for development of more life course-oriented work in social gerontology, and the continued preponderance of gerontological research which focuses on later life rather than the adult life course and the ageing process more widely is reflected in the majority of the chapters.

In tandem with the wider focus of gerontological investigation there has been an expansion of *methodologies* used by the gerontologist. Our book contains examples of the use of new data sources and novel techniques. Hence, included here are chapters considering the use of literature and paintings/photographs as ways of studying ageing and the life course. The use of such cultural products reflects the growing interest in the humanistic approaches and the relevance of cultural studies to gerontology. Our book also takes a closer look at other sources available and at new ways of using these. Thus Victor illustrates different uses of existing data, and Sheridan shows the potential of the Mass-Observation Archive for researchers of ageing. As well as the longitudinal perspective offered by Wadsworth we also have novel uses of methodologies such as diary-based research in gerontology, as shown by Bytheway and Johnson.

Recent years have seen major changes in the *context* within which gerontological research takes place. As the chapter by Gilhooly shows, the ethical context for research, especially that which links to health/social care settings, is now much more complex. All researchers need to be aware of the ethical dimensions of their research. As Netten indicates, this includes all elements of our work, as the research governance framework demonstrates. In the last decade, there has been a growing recognition of the cultural diversity of the ageing experience. In this volume the chapter by Boneham considers the challenges posed when researching ageing in differing cultural contexts.

The chapter by Peace demonstrates the increasingly prominent role of older people in research. Older people are no longer conceptualized as 'passive' recipients of research but as intimately involved in the whole research process. Their involvement is also seen as important in getting research into practice. Nolan and Cook discuss the problems involved in trying to get gerontological research into practice. Having discussed the barriers to the uptake of research they argue for the greater involvement of both practitioners and participants in order to increase the implementation of research.

This volume attempts to reflect the major theoretical and methodological developments in British gerontology over the last two decades. As such it takes a necessarily parochial view and, within a single volume, it is impossible to cover all aspects. We recognize that there is scope for further developments looking at comparative and global aspects of gerontological methodology. Perhaps those will be covered in our next book? We would like to thank all our contributors for their enthusiasm and patience during the preparation of this volume, and the British Society of Gerontology for funding a seminar at which the content and philosophy of the book was shaped.

Reference

Peace, S. (ed.) (1990) *Researching Social Gerontology*. London: Sage Publications.

Part *I*

The who, what and how of social gerontology

1

Theory and practice in social gerontology

Anne Jamieson

The who and where of social gerontology

Gerontology is a multidisciplinary field of study of ageing. It draws on both the physical and social sciences, and, as we shall illustrate in this volume, also includes arts and humanities. Whereas the physical sciences are concerned with the biological aspects of ageing and have a longer tradition, *social gerontology* developed in the mid-1900s as a field of study concerned with ageing in a social context. The boundaries around the social perspectives are to some extent blurred, particularly as regards psychology. Thus the interest in the *individual* experience of ageing, the psychological perspective in *interaction* with the social context, is very much part of social gerontology. We shall return below to the details of what this can mean – the 'what' of social gerontology – and in this section focus on the institutional aspects.

The 'age' dimension has always been part of the interest of social scientists, but usually in a peripheral way, as an 'add-on' dimension in studies where for a long time 'class' was the prime focus, both in theoretical and empirical work. The growing awareness of the demographic changes experienced in the second part of the twentieth century made the older age groups a more obvious focus of attention, and in the last twenty or thirty years the number of researchers engaged in work in the area of gerontology has been growing. Many of these researchers do not necessarily see themselves as 'gerontologists', but as, for example, geographers, economists, sociologists or social policy analysts. They may temporarily be researching ageing issues, or their interest in ageing issues is related to a very specific

aspect or disciplinary perspective. Thus the boundaries around gerontology are not very sharply defined. However, a sizeable proportion of social
researchers have developed a more long-term interest in ageing issues, and,
with it, a broader expertise and understanding of ageing. In this country
many of such researchers would be likely to be members of the British
Society of Gerontology (BSG). This was established in 1971 to provide a
multidisciplinary forum for researchers and others with an interest in promoting the understanding of ageing and later life. It can be seen as part of
the attempt to bring 'age' on to the centre stage of social research. Members
come from a wide range of disciplines, including social policy, sociology,
geography, nursing, social work, psychology, history, social anthropology
and economics. It is a truly multidisciplinary field. This applies not just in
terms of the BSG membership body as a whole, but to a large number of
the individual members, many of whom see themselves as spanning a
range of these disciplines (BSG 1998). It is also reflected in the institutional
affiliations of gerontologists. Most academic gerontologists are based in
departments of sociology, social policy and social work, and various forms
of health studies and medical schools, including geriatric medicine and
nursing. Within the departments, or cutting across departmental/disciplinary
boundaries, there are a number of social (sometimes also including biological and medical) gerontology research centres or institutes. The longest
established ones include the King's College Age Concern Institute of Gerontology; Centre for Gerontology at the University of Keele; the Institute of
Human Ageing at the University of Liverpool; the Centre of Gerontology
and Health Studies at the University of Paisley; and the Centre for Ageing
and Rehabilitation Studies at the University of Sheffield.

The institutional set-up of gerontological research is reflected in the
absence of first degrees purely in gerontology. This is in contrast to the
USA where, in 1999, 203 colleges and universities identified themselves
as offering a bachelor's level programme in gerontology (Kart and Kinney
2001: 537). In the UK, gerontology is seen as a field of study which builds
on the general perspectives and insights of the established social sciences.
The development of social gerontology teaching within universities therefore
has happened in three ways. First, individual courses are offered as part
of undergraduate programmes in subjects such as sociology, social policy,
health studies, including nursing and medicine. Second, a number of universities developed postgraduate Diplomas and Masters programmes in
gerontology. Among the longest established of these are the programmes
at the University of London's King's College and Birkbeck College; the
University of Keele, The Open University, the University of Hull. Third,
short non-degree courses and programmes are offered in a large number
of university settings, aimed primarily to be post-qualifying training and
development for professionals. To use the American terminology (Kart and
Kinney 2001), we are producing 'gerontological specialists', i.e. individuals
who supplement a degree in a traditional discipline with additional training

– as opposed to 'gerontologists', who are defined as those whose training results in a degree in gerontology. Finally, it is worth noting that gerontological training is offered outside the academic institutions, by voluntary organizations such as BASE (British Association for Service to the Elderly).

One of the distinguishing features of many of these gerontology programmes (and indeed, as will be discussed below, of a significant part of research in social gerontology) is their close link to *practice*. Many of the students are engaged in work with older people, most notably in the health and social care sector, although other sectors have become involved more recently, for example through offering retirement preparation programmes for employers.[1] The applied aspect of gerontology is manifest in the fact that research is conducted in a wide variety of settings other than universities, in the statutory, voluntary and private sectors. The close link between research and practice is evident in the constitution of the BSG, which states one of its objectives as being 'the care and relief of the aged'. Many of its members and conference attendees are advocacy groups, professionals and policy makers, seeking research-based evidence and guidance in their work to promote the well-being of older people. How far the research does inform policy and practice is debatable; see Chapter 15 in this volume by Nolan and Cooke.

While the close relation between social gerontology and the practical interest in improving provision of health and social care for older people is thus evident in institutional terms, it should be stressed that the study of *ageing* (as distinct from 'the aged') is not necessarily confined to the study of care-related issues, nor indeed of older people (the definition of whom is in any case problematic). As we shall argue below, it is a much broader field of study, focusing on the processes and dynamics of the adult life course, but, with a few exceptions,[2] this does not appear to be reflected in the teaching programmes around the country.

What is social gerontology?

In trying to identify and describe the – multifaceted and open-ended – field of social gerontology, let us start by raising the following question: what, if anything, binds together this field of thinking and research? In other words, is there a clear research agenda, and what is its rationale? We will seek to answer these questions through an exploration of the theoretical base of the field and its impact on the empirical research.

Theory in gerontology

'Unbearable lightness'?

A recent review by Settersten and Dobransky (2000) of a volume on theory was entitled 'On the unbearable lightness of theory in gerontology' – a wonderful use of a literary allusion, but also a telling description of the per-ception among many gerontologists of the state of their discipline. Thus the view that 'scholarship on aging, at least as it is currently practiced, relegates theory to a position of little or no importance' (Settersten and Dobransky 2000: 367) can be found in much of the literature on gerontology around the world (e.g. Harper 2000; Chappell and Penning 2001; Scharf 2001).

Is theory in gerontology really *'unbearably* light'? In other words, if there is lack of theory, is it a problem? This raises the question of what theory is and what its purpose is. The simplest definition of theory is that it is an *explanation*, an answer to the question why, as distinct from empirical *descriptions*. Theorizing entails reflection as well as empirical observation. The two are not incompatible. The development of theory enables us to understand and make sense of our empirical findings, and also provides us with frameworks and ideas for further research. There is not necessarily a conflict between theoretical aims and *practical* concerns, indeed, it can be argued that the two are inextricably linked (Wilson 2001). In this connec-tion the *critical function* of theory should be emphasized: it can help heighten an awareness of existing biases and practices and develop new ways of understanding the world, transcending existing and dominant discourses. Lack of theory therefore can entail lack of progress in our understand-ing, and a limitation to the value of research (Jamieson and Victor 1997). Anyone setting out to undertake research in a particular area needs to review the field in order to build on what we already know, and not 'reinvent the wheel'. This entails looking for relevant theory, since theory integrates knowledge and provides some clues to the state of our know-ledge in the field.

Does social gerontology suffer from *'lightness* of theory'? Those looking for an overarching 'grand theory' in social gerontology will be disappointed. But then the search for such grand theory has long been abandoned in the social sciences, because it is an aspiration based on a dated positivist view of scientific enterprise as a search for 'universal truths', out there to be discovered. Knowledge is contingent and changeable rather than cumulative. Theoretical developments therefore, in so far as there are any, can be found in the form of *partial theories* on selected aspects of ageing, and in the form of *concepts, frameworks* or *perspectives*. Furthermore, it must be remembered that social gerontology is a *multidisciplinary* field of work, which cannot in itself make claim to be a discipline. The theories in gerontology therefore are most likely to be adapted from or derive from other disciplines.

So, what are the perspectives, what are the relevant disciplines, and what theoretical developments can one discern in this field?

The life course perspective

A key discipline in social gerontology is *sociology*. 'The sociologist', Phillipson argues, is concerned to explore the processes involved and how they are being interpreted by men and women. This approach contrasts with social policy and government interests in old age. In these contexts, old age is regarded as a problem . . . with an emphasis on their similarities [of older people] rather than their differences.

(Phillipson 1998: 5)

So, a sociological starting point does not make any assumptions about the nature of old age. It is important to add that social gerontology is not necessarily confined to studying *old* age, but age more broadly. Riley and Riley talk about the sociology of *age*, which they define as a concern with '(1) people over their life course; (2) age-related social structures and institutions; and (3) the dynamic interplay between people and structures *as each influences the other'* (Riley and Riley 1999: 123). This encapsulates much of what defines social gerontology as a theoretical and empirical field. One should add, however, that the inclusion of *life-span developmental psychology* makes the picture more complete (Blaikie 1992; Sugarman 2001). Thus the challenge of social gerontology as a multidisciplinary field of inquiry is to understand *individual (changing) lives* in the context of *(changing) social structures*, or what others have described as *the life course perspective* (e.g. Hareven 1982). This framework does not specify a particular stage in the life course as the focus. Rather, the focus is on the implications of the passing of *time* for individuals, on the implications and experience of being at a particular point in time, and the links between earlier and later points in time as well as the links between social structures and individual experiences. Although it is not a theory, it defines the field of study from a *theoretical perspective* rather than the perspective of interest groups or policy makers. The dilemma is, however, that the processes and dynamics of adulthood and ageing are complex and difficult to pin down in research; yet, for this very reason, it is important to develop theory to help us identify the important variables and their interrelationships. The life course perspective also has some *methodological implications* (to be discussed in Chapter 2): it highlights the importance of different forms of longitudinal research designs, including life history research.

Much of the (still relatively limited amount of) work undertaken on life course, as distinct from old age issues, comes from outside the UK, mainly the USA (Giele and Elder 1998). It encompasses a broad range of multidisciplinary perspectives, not least social anthropology, where of course there is a long tradition of studying life course transitions (rites of passage). More recently this has been extended to include age concepts more broadly, and the work of Keith *et al.* (1994) comparing age norms and experiences across different cultures is a useful example of the potentials of cross-cultural work in this area. The interest in age norms goes back many decades, with the work of Neugarten *et al.* (1965) often being cited as a key inspiration for later work, including the work of people like Hagestad (1990) and Settersten (1999). For an overview of the work in this field, see Settersten and Mayer (1997). Another focus of work within the life course perspective is upon life events and transitions themselves. In addition to the anthropological work, this has become a key focus in life span developmental psychology (Sugarman 2001), and is a fruitful area for interdisciplinary work and an attempt to integrate individual and social levels of analysis. As Sugarman's book illustrates, although many earlier life span theories can be criticized for their attempt to develop universally applicable models of development, more recent thinking addresses this limitation in its emphasis on diversity and on the ways in which individual lives are socially constructed. The stress on the interconnection in life course research between life span models, like that of Erikson, and broader sociological perspectives is highlighted by Giele and Elder (1998). Their book illustrates well the large amount of work in life course research which has been undertaken for many decades, mainly outside the UK, but also that theoretical development in this field is still modest.

Many social gerontologists would subscribe to the importance of the life course perspective, and to the importance of not confining the field of study to a population defined as 'old' or 'older' through some arbitrary, usually institutionally derived, lower age limit (Peace 1990). Thus many publications have in their titles 'life course' or 'ageing' rather than 'older people' or 'old age' (for example Arber and Evandrou 1993; Bengtson and Schaie 1999). Yet, in practice, even such volumes tend to give weight to issues related to the later years, although a recent exception is Bernard *et al.* (2000a). There is still little material on early or mid-adulthood, and more on the stage of old age than on the processes of ageing. This is perhaps not surprising, because 'it is a complicated endeavour to study the link between individual lives and social change' (Andersson 1999: 134). Yet we would argue that for social gerontology to progress as a theoretically driven field of study, it could benefit from taking a wider life course perspective. As Blaikie (1992: 4) put it,

> Social scientists have been at pains to demonstrate the ways in which class, race and gender permeate the whole of life. In taking for granted the pervasiveness of ageing we have neglected to recognise its full significance as an organising principle that we all of us live with all of the time.

While bearing in mind the need to bring broader life course issues into gerontology, the state of theory in the field relates mainly to the later stage of life. In the following, some of the main developments and debates will be highlighted, but fuller overviews can be found in many introductory gerontology books, such as, for example, Victor (1994) and Kart and Kinney (2001).

Theories, perspectives and research into later life and old age

Individual lives

What does it mean to grow old and to be old? Is it possible to generalize about the experience? Early and still influential theories suggest that it is. One of the first and most fiercely debated theories was *disengagement theory*, put forward by Cumming and Henry (1961). It postulates that society withdraws from the older person to the same extent as the older person withdraws from society, and that therefore there is a functional harmony between the experiences and wishes of older people and those of society. This theory does in fact link the individual and societal levels, and has been criticized at both levels. Thus in contrast to this position is *activity theory*, most often associated with Havighurst (1963), which claims that in order to achieve *successful ageing*, older people need to continue to be active in the same way as they were at middle age. Since these theories were first propounded, they have both been the subject of much criticism, particularly for the way they appear to generalize about *all* older people. Much gerontological work has since attempted to highlight the *diversity* of the ageing experience. This means that research focuses on trying to understand the different factors and circumstances which result in differentiated experiences of later life. One such theory is *continuity theory* (Atchley 1993), which argues that, although people seek change, they also seek a certain amount of continuity, both psychologically and socially. The importance of this theoretical position is evidenced, though not always explicit, in the interest in life histories and the life course perspective. Thus, increasingly, an understanding of people's past is seen as a clue to an understanding of their wishes, feelings and activities in their later lives. Exactly what aspects of people's past matter, and how they influence later life, are questions which are still poorly theorized, although much empirical work is being done. However, the interest in the notion of *successful ageing* or 'productive ageing' has continued, both from psychological and social perspectives. The terms themselves are controversial, and some would reject them as implying some kind of normative vision (Holstein 1999) based on the specific values associated with economic success in capitalist economies. It could be argued, however, that these terms do not necessarily have to assume any judgements on what is 'a good life', and that by deconstructing them it is possible to arrive at alternative interpretations and meanings.

The interest in *meanings* and the meaning of the ageing experience has been growing, and its theoretical roots can be found in a phenomenological – as opposed to a positivist/behaviourist – position (Berger and Luckman 1967). From this perspective, the subjective meanings of the ageing experience, expressed in language and other symbols like paintings and photographs, are considered to be just as real and important to understand as patterns of behaviour. Interpretation and understanding therefore becomes an objective rather than generalizing and theorizing, and the links to the *humanistic* disciplines are evident. In the USA, writers like Cole, Gubrium and Moody are exponents of this approach (Cole *et al.* 1993), along with a number of other 'critical gerontologists'.[3] Thus Gubrium and Wallace (1990: 148) argue that,

> In linking social gerontology and the humanities, scientific theory takes serious consideration of ordinary theorising and draws upon the wide spectrum of experiences, perspectives and interests in developing frameworks . . . In turn, science . . . becomes systematic cultural critique, that is, a professional source of insights for understanding experience, in particular the ageing process.

It is a perspective rather than a theory, a perspective which points in certain directions when it comes to actually doing research. Thus the interest in life stories as told by older people themselves can to some extent be seen to spring from this perspective (see Chapter 2). Similarly, the interest in *images* of ageing and older people, as expressed in art, literature and popular culture, is based on this perspective. In the UK, the work of people like Blaikie and Hepworth figures prominently in this area (see Chapters 3 and 6).

There is one theory which spans the psychological and sociological perspectives and which is the subject of considerable debate: the theory of the *'ageless self'* (Kaufman 1986) or *'the mask of ageing'* (Hepworth 1991). This theory distinguishes between the external, bodily aspects of ageing, and the internal experience of the 'self'. From this theoretical point of view, we remain our young 'selves' while our bodies are marked by the signs of ageing – 'the mask' – with consequences for our social roles. This position is not without its critics (Biggs 1997; Andrews 1999), and the debate about what it really means to grow older continues. It is addressed from a psychological perspective by writers like Biggs (1999) and Coleman (see Chapter 9, this volume), and, as will be discussed below, it is mirrored in sociological thinking (e.g. Gilleard and Higgs 2000) on the meaning of ageing in late modern society.

Structural/macro perspectives: modernity and ageing

Structural or macro analyses focus on the features of society which influence the experience of ageing and later life. An early, and much debated, theory was *modernization theory* (Cowgill and Holmes 1972), which, based on a comparative study of societies at different levels of economic development, drew some general conclusions about the position of older people in modern industrial societies. Their key argument was that, with increasing modernization, the status of older people in the family and in society declines. However, a great deal of evidence has been put forward which throws doubt on the idea of a lost 'golden age' for older people, suggesting that pre-modern societies are complex and variable (e.g. Laslett 1983), and that in modern societies the needs and the contributions of older people are far from ignored by families and the wider community (Twigg and Atkin 1994; Bernard *et al.* 2000b). However, the interest in modernization and its impact on the experience of different life course stages continues to be of central concern, to gerontologists as well as sociologists more generally. Thus the impact of modernization on the development of specific life course stages, and on the new meanings of stages such as adolescence and old age, has been examined by many, for example Hareven (1982), Anderson (1985), and Thane (2000).

The 'modernization' of old age through the development of retirement and the welfare state has been a key focus in social gerontology. Throughout the 1980s one of the most influential theories in Britain was *structural dependency theory* (Townsend 1981) and associated theories (Walker 1981; Phillipson 1982). These theories share a common *political economy* perspective, represented in the USA by writers such as Minkler and Estes (1999) (see Jamieson 2000). This focuses on the ways in which old age is socially constructed by the dominant economic and political interests in capitalist society. Townsend's theory is clear that older people have been made dependent through social policies – which have created poverty among older people and degrading institutionalization and inadequate services for those who are frail. The political economy perspective constitutes a counter attack on the argument in policy circles that the ageing of the population is necessarily bound up with a growing dependency ratio between non-active and working people. It gave rise to a body of research focusing on factors affecting employment and retirement trends (e.g. Kohli *et al.* 1991; Johnson and Falkingham 1992) and poverty and inequalities among older people (see Vincent 1995), both within our own type of society and on a global scale (Wilson 2000). Last, but not least, it provided a theoretical rationale for the already burgeoning interest in the needs of frail old people, the role of the welfare state, and the ways in which service provision dealt with such needs. It has to be said, though, that this vast field of policy-related empirical research is not primarily driven by theory. It is 'deeply rooted in an applied framework . . . with a strong policy focus, reflecting the centrality of governmental funding and concerns, as well as gerontologists' concerns with quality of life as we age' (Chappell and Penning 2001: 100). These comments on Canadian social gerontology apply to the field in most countries, including the USA and UK (Harper 2000; Maddox 2001). While policy- and practice-driven research remains important to practitioners as well as many older people, its dominance in gerontological research has tended to overshadow the development of the theoretical/ conceptual aspects, which are so important if social gerontology is to make a significant contribution to our understanding of ageing in modern society.

Late modernity: social gerontology reconstructed?

Towards the end of the 1980s the structural dependency theory began to be contested as having 'deflected attention away from more progressive and optimistic views of the economic social status of the elderly in modern Britain' (Johnson 1989). This optimistic view of later life is perhaps best encapsulated in Peter Laslett's (1989) 'map of life', a normative vision more than a theory, but representing a clear attempt to conceptualize later life in a more positive way. Thus his map of the four ages, with *'third age'* being the crown of life, reflects the changes experienced for some sections, though by no means all, of the population. It represents a shift in the thinking about the impact of social change on the ageing experience in late modern society. It reflects the changed experiences and *images* of a growing number of older people, the active 'third agers', who have become recognized by business as important *consumers* of a range of commodities such as health and cosmetic products, holidays and retirement homes (Featherstone and Hepworth 1994). A new notion of older people developed, from being products of structural constraints to being social agents, choosing new identities through consumption and lifestyles. Theoretically it represents a renewed emphasis on *agency* within the social context, a 'reconstruction of old age' (Phillipson 1998). Some would still argue that the focus on active lifestyle choices diverts attention from the many forms of social exclusion which still exist in modern societies and globally. Yet social gerontologists generally agree about the *diversity* which exists in the ageing experience, and that any alternative view is ageist. So, if there is such diversity, why not include all possible lives in the realm of social gerontology? Some survey research has highlighted the different forms of social engagement of older people (Midwinter 1991; Sykes and Leather 1997; Walker 1999). But we still know less about the diversity of attitudes and feelings held by older people themselves than about attitudes towards older people. Phillipson (1998) calls for a 'sociology of daily living'. Gilleard and Higgs (2000: 196) call for a more *cuturally orientated* gerontology: 'In place of endless surveil-lance of disability and welfare service utilization', they argue, 'we envisage gerontological social science beginning to pay closer attention to patterns of consumption in later life and to the cohort-based "ageing" of generational lifestyles'. This position could be interpreted as a re-emphasis on the life course perspective, on the need to understand the ageing process, the interaction between agency and (changing) social structures. Thus, for example, the debate about 'the ageless self' can be understood in the context of the development of specific later twentieth-century consumer society, which invites adults to choose their life course strategy, either to attempt to resist ageing or to resist the attempt to remain young. Either strategy is equally real, and both deserve our attention as social gerontologists if we wish to understand the diversity of ageing processes in late modern society.

Social gerontology at the beginning of the twenty-first century has not yet 'come of age'. But it has perhaps reached its stage of turbulent adolescence, turning to new ways of conceptualizing age issues, while still being drawn towards a wish to improve the everyday lives of the most excluded and fragile old people. Funding possibilities from government and other practice-oriented agencies will continue to influence a great deal of gerontological research. Although these are to a large extent geared towards addressing government agendas of the day, research funding councils like the British Economic and Social Research Council (ESRC) offer some potential for social gerontology to combine pressures to conduct 'policy relevant' research with a broader critical function. Its initiative on ageing in the early 1980s contributed a great deal towards the development of a broader research agenda in the UK (Jefferys 1989). Similarly, the more recent 'Growing Older' programme launched in 1999 promises to develop our understanding of the diversity of meanings associated with the notion of 'quality of life' (see GO website in Appendix), although how far it will illuminate issues of *ageing* rather than just *the aged* remains to be seen.

While this chapter has emphasized the importance of theoretical and conceptual work for the development of social gerontology, the remainder of this volume addresses the more practical question of how to go about researching ageing and later life issues, and considers the growing range of strategies and methods available to researchers.

Notes

1 The Pre-Retirement Association is an independent body offering such training programmes.
2 One exception is the MSc in Life Course Development at Birkbeck University of London.
3 For a discussion of 'critical gerontology' in the USA, see Jamieson and Victor 1997 and Jamieson 2000.

References

Anderson, M. (1985) The emergence of the modern life cycle, *Social History*, 10: 1.

Andersson, L. (1999) Sociological research on age: legacy and challenge: a comment, *Ageing and Society*, 19(1): 133–5.

Andrews, M. (1999) The seductiveness of agelessness, *Ageing and Society*, 19: 301–18.

Arber, S. and Evandrou, M. (eds) (1993) *Ageing, Independence and the Life Course*. London: Jessica Kingsley.

Atchley, R.C. (1993) Continuity theory and the evolution of activity in later adulthood, in J.R. Kelly (ed.) *Activity and Ageing*. London: Sage Publications.

Bengtson, V. and Schaie, K.W. (eds) (1999) *Handbook of the Theories of Aging*. New York, NY: Springer.

Berger, P.L. and Luckman, T. (1967) *The Social Construction of Reality*. New York, NY: Anchor Books.

Bernard, M., Phillips, J., Machin, L. and Harding Davies, V. (eds) (2000a) *Women Ageing: Changing Identities, Challenging Myths*. London: Routledge.

Bernard, M., Phillips, J., Phillipson, C. and Ogg, J. (2000b) Continuity and change. The family and community life of older people, in S. Arber and C. Attias-Donfut (eds) *The Myth of Generational Conflict*, pp. 209–27. London: Routledge.

Biggs, S. (1997) Choosing not to be old? Masks, bodies and identity management in later life, *Ageing and Society*, 17: 553–70.

Biggs, S. (1999) *The Mature Imagination*. Buckingham: Open University Press.

Blaikie, A. (1992) Whither the third age? Implications for gerontology, *Generations Review*, 2(1): 2–4.

BSG (British Society of Gerontology) (1998) *Directory of Members' Research Interests and BSG Handbook*. Sheffield: BSG.

Chappell, N.L. and Penning, M. (2001) Sociology of aging in Canada: issues for the millennium, *Canadian Journal on Aging*, 20 (Suppl. 1): 82–110.

Cole, T., Achebaum, W.A., Jacobi, P. and Kastenbaum (eds) (1993) *Voices and Visions of Aging: Toward a Critical Gerontology*. New York, NY: Springer.

Cowgill, D.O. and Holmes, L.D. (1972) *Aging and Modernization*. New York: Appleton-Century-Crofts.

Cumming, E. and Henry, W.E. (1961) *Growing Old*. New York, NY: Basic Books.

Featherstone, M. and Hepworth, M. (1994) Images of ageing, in J. Bond, P. Coleman and S. Peace (eds) *Ageing in Society*, pp. 304–32. London: Sage Publications.

Giele, J.Z. and Elder, G.H. (1998) *Methods of Life Course Research: Qualitative and Quantitative Approaches*. Thousand Oaks, CA.: Sage Publications.

Gilleard, C. and Higgs, P. (2000) *Cultures of Ageing: Self, Citizen and the Body*. London: Prentice-Hall.

Gubrium, J. and Wallace, B. (1990) Who theorises age?, *Ageing and Society*, 10(2): 131–50.

Hagestad, G.U. (1990) Social perspectives on the life course, in R. Binstock and L. George (eds) *Handbook of Aging and the Social Sciences*. New York, NY: Academic.

Hareven, T.K. (1982) The life course and ageing in historical perspectives, in T.K. Hareven and K.J. Adams (eds) *Ageing and Life Course Transitions*. London: Tavistock.

Harper, S. (2000) Ageing 2000 – questions for the 21st century, *Ageing and Society*, 20(1): 111–22.

Havighurst, R.J. (1963) Successful aging, in R.H. Williams, C. Tibbetts and W. Donahue (eds) *Processes of Aging*, pp. 299–320. New York, NY: Atherton.

Hepworth, M. (1991) Positive ageing and the mask of age, *Journal of Educational Gerontology*, 6(2): 93–101.

Holstein, M. (1999) Women and productive aging: troubling implications, in M. Minkler and C.L. Estes (eds) *Critical Gerontology. Perspectives from Political and Moral Economy*. New York, NY: Baywood Publishing Company.

Jamieson, A. (2000) Social gerontology: concepts and concerns in the US and Europe, *European Journal of Social Quality*, 2(1): 88–98.

Jamieson, A. and Victor, C. (1997) Theory and concepts in social gerontology, in A. Jamieson, S. Harper and C. Victor (eds) *Critical Approaches to Ageing and Later Life*. Buckingham: Open University Press.

Jefferys, M. (1989) *Growing Old in the Twentieth Century*. London: Routledge.

Johnson, P. (1989) The structured dependency of the elderly: a critical note, in M. Jefferys (ed.) *Growing Old in the Twentieth Century*, pp. 62–72. London: Routledge.

Johnson, P. and Falkingham, J. (1992) *Ageing and Economic Welfare*. London: Sage Publications.

Kart, C.S. and Kinney, J.M. (2001) *The Realities of Ageing: An Introduction to Gerontology*. Boston: Alan and Bacon.

Kaufman, S. (1986) *The Ageless Self: Sources of Meaning in Late Life*. New York, NY: Meridian.

Keith, J., Fry, C.L., Glascock, A.P. *et al.* (1994) *The Aging Experience*. Thousand Oaks: Sage.

Kohli, M., Rein, M., Guillemard, A.-M. and Gunsteren, H. van (eds) (1991) *Time for Retirement*. Cambridge: Cambridge University Press.

Laslett, P. (1983) *The World we Have Lost – Further Explored*, 3rd edn. London: Methuen.

Laslett, P. (1989) *A Fresh Map of Life*. London: Weidenfeld and Nicolson.

Maddox, G. (2001) Commentary: sociological issues for the millennium, *Canadian Journal on Aging*, 20 (Suppl. 1): 111–17.

Midwinter, E. (1991) *The British Gas Report on Attitudes to Ageing 1991*. London: British Gas.

Minkler, M. and Estes, C.L. (eds) (1999) *Critical Gerontology. Perspectives from Political and Moral Economy*. New York, NY: Baywood Publishing Company.

Neugarten, B.L., Moore, J.W. and Lowe, J.C. (1965) Age norms, age constraints and adult socialization, *American Journal of Sociology*, 70: 710–17.

Peace, S. (1990) Introduction: researching social gerontology: concepts, methods and issues, in S. Peace (ed.) *Researching Social Gerontology*. London: Sage Publications.

Phillipson, C. (1982) *Capitalism and the Construction of Old Age*. London: Macmillan.

Phillipson, C. (1998) *Reconstructing Old Age*. London: Sage Publications.

Riley, M.W. and Riley, J.W. (1999) Sociological research on age: legacy and challenge, *Ageing and Society*, 19(1): 123–32.

Scharf, T. (2001) Social gerontology in Germany: historical trends and recent developments, *Ageing and Society*, 21(4): 489–505.

Settersten, R.A. (1999) *Lives in Time and Place: The Problems and Promises of Developmental Science*. Amityville, NY: Baywood Publishing Company.

Settersten, R.A. and Dobransky, L.M. (2000) On the unbearable lightness of theory in gerontology, *The Gerontologist*, 40(3): 367–73.

Settersten, R.A. and Mayer, K.U. (1997) The measurement of age, age structuring and the life course, *Annual Review of Sociology*, 23: 233–61.

Sugarman, L. (2001) *Life-Span Development*. Hove: Taylor & Francis.

Sykes, R. and Leather, R. (1997) *Grey Matters: A Survey of Older People in England*. London: Anchor Trust.

Thane, P. (2000) *Old Age in English History*. Oxford: Oxford University Press.

Townsend, P. (1981) The structured dependency of the elderly: a creation of social policy in the twentieth century, *Ageing and Society*, 1(1): 5–28.

Twigg, J. and Atkin, K. (1994) *Carers Perceived: Policy and Practice in Informal Care*. Buckingham: Open University Press.

Victor, C. (1994) *Old Age in Modern Society*. London: Chapman and Hall.

Vincent, J.A. (1995) *Inequality and Old Age*. London: UCL Press.

Walker, A. (1981) Toward a political economy of old age, *Ageing and Society*, 1(1): 73–94.

Walker, A. (ed.) (1999) *The Politics of Old Age in Europe*. Buckingham: Open University Press.

Wilson, G. (2000) *Understanding Old Age. Critical and Global Perspectives*. London: Sage Publications.

Wilson, G. (2001) Conceptual frameworks and emancipatory research in social gerontology, *Ageing and Society*, 21(4): 471–87.

2

Strategies and methods in researching ageing and later life

Anne Jamieson

Age, period and cohort

In some respects, the practical research issues related to social gerontology are little different from those in other areas of social research, and a large number of books on generic social research methodologies are on the market, at both introductory and advanced levels.[1] However, there are some research issues which are specific to the study of ageing, and there are strategies and methodologies which are particularly suited to social gerontology inquiry.[2] The contributions to this volume aim to illustrate the ways in which different sources and methods can be used specifically to throw light on relevant questions in this field.

As argued in Chapter 1, the focus of social gerontology is upon the under-standing of individual (changing) lives in the context of (changing) social structures. Central is the passing of *time*, both for individuals ('individual time') and for society (historical time). This (life course) perspective pre-sents some challenging methodological issues to the researcher. It is often referred to as the 'age/period/cohort (APC) problem'. The issue is one of distinguishing between changes which are a function of individual matura-tion (age effects), and changes which are due to the impact of social factors (period and cohort effects). Thus, differences found through cross-sectional comparisons of characteristics of different age groups (cohorts) could be due to the different social contexts in which they have been developing rather than their chronological age and are described as cohort effects. These differences would manifest themselves in future social change, as the younger generations grow older and replace the current older generations. Social influences that affect all cohorts or generations at a given time are referred to as 'period effects'. They represent general social change and will of course also influence the changes observed in individuals as they go through the life course. The more we understand about the factors affecting individual ageing/life course changes, the more we would be able to understand the implications for present and future social relations. Conversely, a better understanding of social change will help the development of insight into individual life courses and experiences of specific life course stages. In the following we shall consider the different research strategies included in this volume,[3] in relation to these two different (but very much interconnecting) levels of analysis.

Individual lives

Processes of change

The focus on individual *ageing* is associated with a number of questions such as: what changes occur to individuals as they pass through time, in terms of health, abilities, attitudes, activities and social relations? In what ways does the social context affect such changes, and to what extent are they related to chronological age? To what extent and in what ways do earlier life course experiences affect experiences, opportunities, resources and social relations in later life? In theoretical terms (see Chapter 1), one of the central questions is how far and in what ways continuity theory applies.

Simple cross-sectional comparisons of different age groups do not necessarily tell us about change processes. For this *longitudinal approaches* have greater potential. Such approaches encompass a range of different strategies, although the term longitudinal is most commonly associated with *prospective* longitudinal work – follow-up studies – whereby data are collected about the same individuals *at* different points in time (see Wadsworth, Chapter 7). However, information relating to individuals *about* different points in time can also be collected *retrospectively*, relying on recall, and such studies are usually referred to as *life history* or *biographical approaches* (see Bornat, Chapter 8). Combinations of retrospective and prospective studies are possible, for example in *catch-up designs*, whereby individuals from a previous study are traced and studied at a later time, either as a one-off follow-up study or combined with further prospective study. The time period over which individuals are studied can vary considerably. Many longitudinal studies initiated by gerontologists focus on the later years of the life course, following individuals through from early to late old age, for example Coleman's twenty-year longitudinal study of older people (see Chapter 9). But many studies which were not set up specifically to understand ageing start as early as the time of birth. In Britain there are several such birth cohort studies, including the 1946 birth cohort study directed by Wadsworth (see Chapter 7). The subjects in this study are now in their fifties, and it will need quite a few years' worth of follow-up studies before we can draw the full benefits of this work. However, it already tells us a great deal about the adult life course and about the interaction between biological and social factors over the life course in regard to health and social relations. The study has gathered information about a wide range of social factors, including life events, and their subsequent impact, for example the impact of parental divorce on children's educational performance. Furthermore, as Wadsworth points out, through these studies of 'developmental processes and experiences in the years before later life begins, it is increasingly possible to anticipate some important features of the later life of future generations' (p. 113). While a longitudinal study allows one to follow the same individuals over time, exploring the interplay between biological, psychological and social factors, the results are not necessarily generalizable, as there may be hidden cohort effects. However, it is possible to overcome this by comparing results from different cohort studies, of which there are a growing number.

Prospective longitudinal studies are not without their problems and limitations, as illustrated by Wadsworth. Furthermore, large-scale, long-term birth cohort studies are not very feasible for individuals to embark on. For researchers who do not have the resources and who wish to have results rather more quickly, *retrospective studies* are a more realistic option. *Life history research* (see Chapter 8) offers the opportunity to get information about people's lives, *as they recollect* them. Although life history or biographical studies tend to be small-scale and apply qualitative analyses, and prospective longitudinal studies tend to be large-scale studies analysed quantitatively, in principle prospective as well as retrospective studies could be both quantitative and qualitative,[4] see Coleman in this volume, and Dex (1991). In practice, the life history tradition emphasizes in-depth qualitative research. Indeed, as Bornat argues, it is seen as one of its strengths that in many studies older people are allowed and encouraged to determine the agenda for the research process, telling *their* story and raising points that are important to them. Thus it may throw light on forgotten or hidden aspects of past experience, and highlight minority experiences, which tend to be hidden in more quantitative studies. Of course, life history interviews can be structured, so that information about specific aspects of earlier life can be explored with a view to understanding later life. Although relying on people's own constructions of the past can have its advantages in alerting the researcher to new interpretations, there can of course also be disadvantages. Thus the stories people tell are affected not only by what they can recall, but also by how they choose to interpret these memories. In some cases it is possible to triangulate data (see Kellaher *et al.* 1990) and compare people's oral stories with other sources of information. This is emphasized by

Coleman (Chapter 9), whose discussion of *psychobiographical work* complements the sociologists' interests in biographies, and suggests that in combination they can offer an important way forward in understanding the ageing process as the interaction between individual change and social change. His own empirical work is interesting in the sense that his methodology combines a quantitative longitudinal study with in-depth qualitative analysis. The latter has not been looked upon very favourably within mainstream psychology, which emphasizes quantitative work and the importance of generalizability of research findings. But there are encouraging signs that more small-scale, qualitative studies is becoming more acceptable. Case studies, although in themselves not generalizable, can be used to generate hypotheses and to test existing theory at the level of the individual. Furthermore, case studies can add more illuminative aspects to large-scale studies.

Experiences in later life: choices, constraints and strategies

Most empirical research in social gerontology focuses on later life, or 'older people', and, as discussed in Chapter 1, some of the recent theoretical debates focus on what constitute the sources of identity in old age, and on how far older individuals are adopting a wider range of active strategies for coping with and enjoying later life.

Much of the life history research already mentioned is used to explore the lives of older people, and in some contexts the question of whether the memories are 'correct' is seen as less relevant than what they express about the present state of the older person. (For the use of memories for this purpose, see Fairhurst 1997.)

But there is a range of other sources and methods for exploring the lives of older people. One method is the use of *diaries*. Historians use diaries, kept by individuals for their own reasons, and the Mass-Observation Archive (see below) also collects diaries. Some of these are constructed in response to specific concerns, such as food habits. The use of commissioned as distinct from purely personal diaries in social research is still relatively rare, although becoming more popular. It would seem a particularly fruitful option for social gerontologists, both because diaries are about use of *time* and because they can be a useful *aide memoire* for people whose memory may be less sharp. They can be a way of gaining access both to what actually happens and to the subjective meanings attributed to such events. Bytheway and Johnson (Chapter 10) report in detail on their own use of diaries in understanding how older people manage their long-term medication. In this case highly structured diary templates were used, and they were complemented by interviews. Diaries can reveal insight into the complex patterns of daily routines and social relations. As with any method, there are limitations and disadvantages. Having to record things in writing can put some people off for a variety of reasons, for example the fear of being incompetent, poor eyesight or lack of energy. To some extent this can be overcome by the use of scribes, but, depending on the topics explored, this may influence the results. On the other hand, many of the participants in Bytheway and Johnson's study did in any case keep journals or diaries of some nature, which raises the question of whether there might be some untapped potential for researchers in this area.

The Mass-Observation Archive, described by Sheridan (Chapter 5), represents an interesting and unusual source for researchers. Launched in the 1930s to document everyday life as described by 'ordinary people' themselves, it was revived in the 1980s and continues to this day. The archive consists of diaries and responses to specific 'directives', covering a wide range of social issues, submitted by volunteers. The fact that the contributors are self-selected individuals, who are specifically motivated and able to express themselves in writing, clearly imposes limitations on the extent to which generalizations can be made. Also, although responding to directives, contributors themselves control the agenda and what they write. This may limit the extent of comparability between cases, but, as with open-ended life history interviews, it can be seen as a strength for certain purposes that the material is not constructed through a particular research tool. Furthermore, its preponderance of older people, yet with the inclusion of other age groups, means that there is potential to compare age groups in terms of attitudes and lifestyle in a range of areas. Furthermore, because some have been contributing over many years, it is possible to analyse individual change.

Gerontologists of the ethnomethodological tradition (see Chapter 1), whose concern is to understand what it *means* to grow old and the diversity of meanings and subjective experiences attached to ageing, have long had a particular interest in cultural products, particularly fiction. Literary gerontology, as Hepworth explains (Chapter 6), started to develop in the 1970s, and has been particularly popular in the USA, where the humanistic approach has been promoted as an alternative to the more positivist, so-called scientific perspectives. Cultural research challenges us to understand the problematic nature of all knowledge. 'Facts' and 'fiction' are both culturally constructed, and, as Hepworth points out, science 'borrows' from the wider culture metaphors and images of ageing. Fiction deals with many of the important issues in social gerontology, like changes in intimate relations over the life course, sexuality, family conflict, loss and death. Many of these very private topics are difficult to research in conventional ways, and novels and short stories can explore the emotional, some would add spiritual, aspects of individual experiences. The theoretical base for much literary gerontology, including Hepworth's work, is symbolic interactionism (see Chapter 1). He gives two examples of his literary analysis, both from popular crime fiction, and illustrates how such analyses can unveil diverse images of ageing, help us understand the variations in the ageing experience and promote new agendas for positive ageing. As with much other material, there are issues of representativeness and therefore the validity of fiction as a source. It is crucial therefore to analyse fictional accounts in the context of conventional gerontological knowledge. The humanistic disciplines are complementary and do not replace scientific inquiry, but they would seem to be highly relevant in the development of a more culturally oriented gerontology (see Chapter 1).

With the expansion of the mass media, whether newspapers, magazines, TV or the Internet, the range of cultural products at the disposal of social researchers in today's society has become almost overwhelming. All around us are images and stories of adulthood, ageing and old age. While they constitute a potential source for gerontological researchers, the problems of selection and representativeness have not become any easier than for researchers of the past.

Social trends and social change

The past and the process of modernization

Questions related to the ways in which the experience of ageing and attitudes to old age have changed, for example as expressed in modernization theory, continue to occupy historians and social gerontologists. The methods available in this area are different. Those wishing to research the past are by definition confined to analyses of existing sources, and, as Blaikie points out in Chapter 3, the more distant the past, the less the range of sources available. The most recent past presents more possibilities, including the possibility of talking to survivors, as witnessed in the increasingly popular oral history tradition (see Bornat, Chapter 8). Whatever the sources from the past, whether pictures, fiction, diaries or records, there are important issues both of *representativeness* and of the *meaning* of the material. For example, was Ariès (1962) right in his conclusions about the absence of childhood before the sixteenth century, which he drew from considering paintings of the period? Or did he base his view on a misinterpretation of the paintings, which in any case were perhaps not representative of life in general? Whether pictures, text or statistics, the behaviour recorded in the past may have had specific meanings which are inaccessible to the present-day researcher. Blaikie discusses two examples of work using existing sources. The first concerns social surveys conducted between the 1890s and the 1940s, a period much less researched than earlier and later periods. Blaikie assesses the usefulness of these sources in throwing light on the social circumstances of older people in poverty. He illustrates how uneven the information is and therefore how difficult it is to obtain anything like a comprehensive view of the question. The second example is an analysis of photographs, which constitute an interesting source for the study of stereotypical images since the late nineteenth century. Blaikie discusses photographs from particular localities (East Coast fishing communities) in a specific period (1850–1914). He highlights the growing range of photographic archives available for scrutiny, including websites, but also urges a notion of caution against drawing general conclusions from such images, and emphasizes the importance of considering the context within which they were constructed and selected for the archives.

Recent trends and current diversities

The more recent the past we are interested in, the more information is available. The Mass-Observation Archive has already been mentioned, and it is in some respects possible to explore questions of cohort change by comparing material from the 1930s with more recent material. During the twentieth century data processing technology has been revolutionized, and modern societies have become 'data rich'. Victor (Chapter 4) considers the many different existing sets of statistical data which are available in the form of government and other publications as well as archives of raw data. With the new web technology, researchers are able to access a wide range of information easily and cheaply. But, as for the sources discussed by Blaikie, the purpose for which they were compiled is usually different from the research in hand. Thus secondary analysis is defined as the reanalysis and interpretation of research data which were originally collected for a different purpose and/or by other researchers. This is indeed the limitation of using existing data, and the attraction for researchers in collecting their own data is the apparent control they can exercise in the information they collect. However, in reality this control is usually severely curtailed by practical and financial constraints, and often secondary analysis can provide much better value for money. Regular major surveys can yield a great deal of relevance to questions related to a range of activities and attitudes of different age cohorts, and can also be used to trace changes over time. Information on the current characteristics of middle-aged and older people, e.g. on employment, inequalities and social exclusion, on consumption patterns and attitudes, goes some way towards illuminating the theoretical issues around the role of older people in today's society. Anyone contemplating new data collection would be wise at least to consult existing published statistics. Such data can be useful for giving a broad picture of representative samples of the population and form the context for smaller scale studies.

Social policy and practice

As mentioned in Chapter 1, social policy issues, including care needs and service provision, constitute a large part of social gerontological inquiry.

This volume focuses primarily on the broader sociological issues of ageing and later life experiences. But many of these do of course have relevance to social policy debates: for example, the structural dependency theory is pointing at social policies as the origin of the situation of older people. Also, studies of older people's daily lives can be directly related to issues of service provision, as demonstrated by Bytheway and Johnson's use of diaries.

The study reported by Bytheway and Johnson was funded by *service providers*, in their case the Department of Health, seeking information on how older people manage long-term medication. A large amount of research is undertaken which aims to help improve services and other interventions like drugs treatment, for older people, using a variety of methods, including those discussed above. Studies may be more or less directly related to service provision; at one end of the spectrum studies could focus on older people's activities and social relations, including care needs and care commitments, aimed to throw light on their needs and assess the adequacy of existing provision. At the other end of the spectrum is research focusing on very specific interventions and their effectiveness. These are the *evaluation studies* discussed by Netten (Chapter 11). There is a range of designs and approaches to evaluation, and a great deal of literature already exists on this topic. However, in many studies, the measures and criteria used in assessing services are not necessarily geared to take into account the situation of older people, with the result that conclusions can be ageist. It is important for those embarking on such research, whether in health or in social service evaluation, to be aware of these issues. Netten discusses details of an evaluation study related to the Care in the Community Programme. A key concern in this kind of study is with what could be described in simple terms as *value for money*. In other words, for service funders the economic aspects of the evaluation are crucial. But, as Netten illustrates, there are many methodological challenges associated with identifying both outcomes of interventions and true costs. Thus, short of using controlled experiments as in drug trials, because they are often both impractical and unethical, alternative methods raise problems of establishing causal relations between 'input' and outcome. On the cost side, there are also difficulties in developing exact measures, for example when it comes to assessing the costs to informal carers in the form of time and stress. Netten draws many lessons from her case study, which are useful even for those embarking on smaller scale evaluation studies.

Research methods compared

To many, the distinction between 'using existing sources' and 'creating new data' raises the question of what original research is. Originality, or progress in our understanding, lies in the way the world is analysed and conceptualized. The process of 'going out there' and interviewing people is sometimes seen as the epitome of original research, but a questionnaire or interview survey asking dull questions can yield some very uninteresting, unoriginal results. Imaginative and rigorous analyses of existing texts, data, photos or stories can make contributions to the field which are just as original, sometimes more so. There are several attractions to collecting fresh material from individuals through, for example, field work, interviews and questionnaire surveys. Thus, although collecting and processing new data can be extremely time-consuming for academics working in the university sector it can provide opportunities for them to obtain research grants to hire assistants, and thereby help improve their university's research rating![5] There are, of course, more important reasons for creating new data. The main attraction is in the degree of control that can apparently be exercised by the researcher over whom to study and what to ask. In practice this control is, of course, curbed by a wide range of factors such as access and willingness and ability of potential respondents to cooperate.

In reviewing the range of strategies and methods available to the researcher, it should be obvious that, apart from personal preferences and financial considerations, choices of what are the most appropriate methods are in large part dependent on one's initial questions or aims. The contributions in this volume illustrate that there is a wide range of research questions and methods, which also represent – sometimes implicitly – a variety of positions regarding the meaning and purpose of research. Thus there is a distinction between, on the one hand, so-called nomothetic research aimed at generalization and explanation and therefore theory, and, on the other hand, ideographic research, aimed at description and meanings of unique occurrences. The former is most often associated with large-scale quantitative measurements, whereas the latter, humanistic approach tends to entail in-depth interpretation of sources, whether written or spoken, as in literature, arts and history. Coleman (Chapter 9) quotes Murray, who said 'every person is in certain respects like all other persons, like some other persons, and like no other persons' (p. 36).

This quote, it seems to us, illustrates why we need different types of research. A single case or a few cases, whether chosen from a diary from the past, a novel, a case study or biography, has the potential of teaching us something about the experience of adulthood and ageing, either by illuminating the familiar, or by highlighting the unfamiliar, thus yielding new ideas and concepts. But we also need to explore broader commonalities of experience and to unveil patterns of diversity.

The roles and responsibilities of the researcher

A distinction is often made between two contrasting, ideal type, research paradigms (see Peace, Chapter 14), i.e. the *positivist* and the *emancipatory* paradigms. One of the features claimed to distinguish so-called positivist researchers is their view of *the role of the researcher*. Thus the positivist sees the researcher as separate from the research subjects, observing them as objects like a scientist. In many ways this is a caricature of a bad researcher, and most good social researchers would be aware of the role of the subjects in the research process, and the ways in which this process might affect them. Indeed, there has been a growing awareness of the ethical aspects of research. Gilhooly (Chapter 13), in her discussion of ethical issues, lists four overriding guiding principles, which are: do no harm (non-maleficence); do positive good (beneficence); show respect for people's autonomy; and treat people fairly. In her chapter the notions of consent, confidentiality and privacy are discussed, as are the institutional aspects relating to the monitoring of ethical aspects. For anyone embarking on empirical research, it is essential to be aware of the minimal requirements for ethically acceptable research, and increasingly this is being monitored and governed in institutions undertaking research, whether in the National Health Service (NHS) or in universities (Tinker 2001).

In recent years, many social gerontologists have begun to extend the responsibility of researchers to include the *involvement of older people* in the research process itself. This, as Peace points out in Chapter 14, can be seen in the context of a general move, at least in the rhetoric, towards democratization and involvement of ordinary people in community affairs, and it relates to the ethical principle, mentioned by Gilhooly, of beneficence ('doing positive good'). It has its roots in the school of thinking, evident in feminist research, which emphasizes the importance of the personal commitment of the researcher to empower socially weak groups. In the context of social gerontology, these issues have become particularly pertinent in the area of directly applied research into service provision. 'Involvement' can mean many things, from consulting users about what kind of research they deem most appropriate, to actually engaging them in all aspects of the research process from design and data collection to analysis. This raises questions of the representativeness of those who become involved, and of their abilities to undertake and influence research. Above all, it raises the question of whether the research itself will be better and more useful. Boneham (Chapter 12) gives examples of how her research into the needs of certain ethnic minority communities would be almost futile without the active involvement of representatives from these communities. This was not only for reasons of access and communication, but also in order to understand what really concerned some of these minority groups. Through an action research approach it became possible to disclose some of the myths surrounding certain minority groups, for example the myth that families look after each other and services are not needed.

It is possible to see the relation between researchers and the 'researched' on a continuum of involvement and power, ranging from one of complete detachment (for example as respondents to a postal questionnaire), to one in which the researched or their representatives are collaborators with the researchers throughout the research process. In between these extremes are variations, such as the respondents to the Mass-Observation Archive, or participants in open-ended life history interviews. Anyone embarking on a piece of empirical research should think through the role of their 'research objects', be they younger or older, service users or providers, and consider this in relation to their specific research aims. Training a handful of older people to be the interviewers in a project can in some circumstances serve a useful purpose. But in other situations this may be no more than some token involvement, at best useless and at worst harmful to both the older people and the research process.

The rationale underlying the efforts of many somehow to involve not only older people, but practitioners, is the wish for the research to 'be useful'. Nolan and Cooke (Chapter 15) discuss the problems associated with making research of practical use. There is much talk in public policy, in areas such as health and social services and education, of the need for evidence-based practice, and there is no doubt that practices could be improved by the availability and use of relevant research. Nolan and Cooke discuss the many barriers to the implementation of evidence-based practice, which relate not only to the nature of the research undertaken, but problems of dissemination and adoption. This raises the question of whether the distinction commonly made between theoretical, empirical and applied research is actually meaningful. Clearly, research that is categorized as 'applied' does not always get used, and research aimed primarily at developing insight and explanations can very well be 'useful' and affect practices in a broader sense of the term.

Undoubtedly there continues to be a need for researchers to devote efforts to solving the practical problems of today, to improve the conditions for the frailest older people, and to influence policy and practice in this area. However, as we hope to illustrate in this volume, there are other agendas for researchers in social gerontology. As an area of study it needs to address the wider issues associated with ageing in the twenty-first century. This means going beyond a focus on the needs and frailties of old people, and, as argued in Chapter 1, exploring the different cultures of ageing which have emerged. Such foci, while having the potential of developing social gerontology as a serious field of study, do not necessarily entail a distancing of research from practice. Social gerontology, as other social sciences, has a critical role to perform in society, although interpretations of what that means will no doubt vary between researchers, as the contributions to this volume illustrate.

Notes

1 Any search for literature on research methods will yield a vast array of choices. The preferred choices will depend not only on the experience of the individual

researcher but on the specific methodologies the researcher plans to use. For a basic and clear introductory book, see Denscombe (1998).

2 Terms like approach, strategy and method are often used interchangeably. Denscombe (1998) distinguishes between different strategies and methods. Strategies include surveys, case studies, experiments, action research and ethnography. Methods refer to use of questionnaires, interviews, observation and documents.

3 The contributions to this volume encompass a wide range of different strategies and methods, but do not cover everything possible. Among the most obvious omissions are observation and *ethnographic studies*. These have been used in settings where older people get together, such as clubs and day centres, not only to consider service use, but also to explore broader issues related to social relations among older people, e.g. Hazan (1980). However, the use of ethnography in exploring processes in service settings is particularly pertinent; see Fairhurst (1997) for an account of its use in a hospital unit. Another growing area of research is the area of cross-national comparison. The very pertinent research issues in this area are not included in this book.

4 The distinction between quantitative and qualitative research is, strictly speaking, a distinction in terms of method of *analysis* rather than data collection. Thus quantitative methods can be used on textual material (content analysis), and large-scale surveys can have open-ended questions which could be analysed qualitatively rather than in terms of numbers.

5 Ray Pahl (1995) in his book *After Success* has a rather witty appendix on 'Method', in which he describes how the book was written with very little funding support. He goes on, 'However, the *cognoscenti* of social science research will recognise a disaster when they see one. I brought no outside funds to the university; I employed no research assistants and did not have to pay for interviewers, coders and data processing and analysis' (p. 201).

References

Ariès, P. (1962) *Centuries of Childhood*. London: Jonathan Cape.

Denscombe, M. (1998) *The Good Research Guide*. Buckingham: Open University Press.

Dex, S. (ed.) (1991) *Life and Work History Analyses: Qualitative and Quantitative Developments*. London: Routledge.

Fairhurst, E. (1997) Recalling life: analytical issues in the use of 'memories', in A. Jamieson, S. Harper and C. Victor (eds) *Critical Approaches to Ageing and Later Life*. Buckingham: Open University Press.

Hazan, H. (1980) *The Limbo People. A Study in the Constitution of the Time Universe among the Aged*. London: Routledge and Kegan Paul.

Kellaher, L., Peace, S. and Willcocks, D. (1990) Triangulating data, in S. Peace (ed.) *Researching Social Gerontology*. London: Sage Publications.

Pahl, R. (1995) *After Success*. Cambridge: Polity Press.

Tinker, A. (2001) Ethics commitees – help or hindrance?, *Generations Review*, 11(3): 11–12.

Part *II*

Using existing sources

3

Using documentary material: researching the past

Andrew Blaikie

Introduction

Historical analysis must address three fundamental issues: the questions one wishes to ask; the sources that are available; and the methods by which to investigate the data. These matters are interrelated in that the possibilities for studying old age in the past are in high degree determined by the availability and nature of documentary evidence. Original data concerning the ancient world consist of material such as hieroglyphs, biblical texts, Greek tragedies, Icelandic sagas and paintings. In a largely pre-literate epoch, only the powerful recorded their thoughts (Finley 1984; Parkin 1998). However, the emergence of bureaucracies, first local and ecclesiastical, latterly national and secular, gave rise to more socially inclusive information such as parish registers, inventories and Poor Law ledgers (Pelling and Smith 1991), then to more comprehensive pensions information in the twentieth century (Johnson 1985; Hannah 1986; Hunt 1989). Textual sources reflecting the views of elites in the distant past are not comparable with surveys of pensioners in recent times. And they are certainly distinct from, say, oral narratives recorded in the last thirty years. Scholars of ageing at different periods have accordingly adopted differing emphases, those considering the deep past focusing upon cultural representations as evidenced in art, or the prescriptive literatures of medicine and religion, while analyses of pre-industrial society have considered demographic issues such as population ageing and the detailed composition of the household (Laslett 1977; Wall 1984; Minois 1989).

Nevertheless, similar questions have been asked of widely varying sources since, arguably, gerontological thought has been obsessed with an overarching debate over the impact of modernization on societal attitudes towards the aged (Achenbaum and Stearns 1978; Troyansky 1997; Johnson and Thane 1998; Thane 2000). On the one hand, the supposed effects of the Industrial Revolution have prompted a before-versus-after argument in which a lost 'golden age of senescence' has been replaced by a dark era of dependency and disdain; on the other, this characterization has been questioned by a stance emphasizing ongoing ambiguities and 'co-existent competing conceptions' of older people during each period (Thane 1995: 31). The very existence of this debate testifies to the difficulty of providing conclusive documentary evidence to support either proposition. Key themes covered in the literature include: respect for elders versus degradation of the aged; structured dependency versus autonomy; intergenerational harmony versus conflict; and diversity versus homogeneity of attitudes and behaviour towards older people (Thomas 1977; Townsend 1981; Smith 1984; Johnson *et al.* 1989; Thane 1995). Rather than engage further in historiographic debate, this chapter focuses on some methodological issues involved in analysing specific types of documentary material pertaining to relatively recent times. First, however, it is useful to note a number of considerations that apply to all historical data.

Representation and meaning

The researcher must begin by asking: how reliable are the sources I am using? Historical sources tend to be locally as well as temporally specific, thus difficult to interpret out of their unique context. If we are to avoid drawing gross generalizations from data that may be far from typical we have to subject our sources to a range of tests for representativeness. Moreover, it is usually necessary to take samples, either because of the sheer volume of material (e.g. the census), or due to the paucity of information; there may be only one or two shreds of highly atypical evidence from which to select (e.g. literary attitudes to older women in ancient Rome). In each instance, we must justify the grounds on which we have chosen our data. A key question will be: what other evidence do I have to compare my source with?

The French historian Philippe Ariès has argued that before the sixteenth century there was no concept of childhood in Western Europe and that all persons aged 7 and above were regarded as miniature adults (Ariès 1962). He bases his argument on the paintings of the period. He could be right, but critics have suggested that he may just as easily be wide of the mark (Wilson 1980). The problem is that, graphic though the details of the portraits may be, the imagery of young persons may reflect an artistic fashion, rather than an attempt at realism; second, they might instance the personal style or whim of the artist; and third, even supposing they are realistic, the only people who were painted were those who could afford to be, and their treatment of children could scarcely be held up as representative of society as a whole.

By the same token, it is necessary to be circumspect in our interpretation of images of later life. Were we to study, say, Rembrandt's portraits of older people (including himself) we would have to ask similar questions. In his sketches of heads preparatory to his 'A Portrait of a Lady Aged Sixty-Two' (1632), the artist exaggerated wrinkles for picturesque effect, but in the finished portrait they have disappeared – instead her skin is 'delicately creased, her gaze sparkles with a fine line of white along a lower eyelid, and her apple cheeks are smooth'. Similarly, by 1655 his 'An Old Woman Reading' indicates

> how Rembrandt developed and refined such depictions of old women over the years . . . though others sometimes depicted the elderly as decrepit and foolish, Rembrandt shows them as 'waiting, meditating and reading, taking on a profound human dignity through their faith and hope'.
>
> (National Galleries of Scotland 2001)

This problem applies to qualitative textual materials such as diaries, newspapers, novels and memoirs, for in each case we are looking the wrong way through the telescope and into the eye of the beholder (Laslett 1976). What we must do is understand the socially specific context in which the works were produced by subjecting our information to inference tests. Consider the example of the oft-quoted speech by Jaques in Shakespeare's *As You Like It* (Act II, Scene VII), which summarizes the nature of each age of man, ending with 'last scene of all . . . second childishness and mere oblivion, sans teeth, sans eyes, sans taste, sans everything' (Shakespeare 1906: 227). Assessing the veracity of this observation as representative of Elizabethan old age requires us first to ask whether Shakespeare was in a position of first-hand knowledge. He was 35 when he wrote the play, and thus unlikely to be particularly sympathetic or knowledgeable about the experience of later life. Secondly, we should consider the literary context: the characters are not situated in real time but in a mythical pastoral. Without corroboration from other sources, it is impossible to judge whether or not the observation of a fictional melancholic lord (Jaques) finds salience with typical contemporary perceptions, still less whether his remark reflected reality. Since Jaques's speech is followed by the stage entrance of a 'strong and lusty' octogenarian, we have to assume that Shakespeare's sense of the properties of later life was ambiguous (Thane 2000: 7), as well as his sense of earlier life. Juliet marries Romeo at age 13. However, demographers have discovered that the mean age at first marriage in Elizabethan England was around 25, and in Italy much the same.

For pre-industrial and modern times, using quantitative records becomes increasingly feasible. However, further problems of representativeness arise. All sources are socially constructed and official policy documents, censuses and surveys present no exception. The researcher must consider problems of definition and classification. For example, under the Old Poor Law (before 1834), the term 'pensioner' applied to those relieved not only on grounds of age but also according to disability, while the amount of pension given to each individual varied massively (Laslett 1989: 128). The judgement of these criteria varied considerably between parishes and over time. Thus to apply the current, nationally comprehensive and rigid usage to historical data would be misleadingly anachronistic while comparative studies require a prior understanding of the varying evaluations of local officials.

Much of what is written about ageing, including official policy documents, was written with a polemical aim in mind and needs to be understood as such (Thane 2000: 6). Sometimes this is obvious, as, for example, with a report title like *The Impending Crisis of Old Age* (Shegog 1981). But more often biases are hidden behind the production of apparently objective statistics (Hindess 1973). Problems of meaning always occur when quantitative observations are used to interpret social behaviour. Hence it becomes necessary to consider why a particular survey was conducted or why records were originally kept, particularly since the reasons for collecting information then usually differ from the reasons why we wish to read it now. With large collections there is also the issue of 'weeding' to consider: what proportion of the original source was retained and on what basis were the samples selected?

Second, and more significant, is the question of what the behaviour recorded generally meant to contemporaries. On the basis of statistics from census and other listings demographers often cite the widespread distribution and long-term endurance of the nuclear-household system as a key characteristic of the Western family system. However, this formal observation fails to acknowledge the variability of attitudes which probably existed within the nuclear household, and which was arguably of far greater importance. As Anderson remarks,

> To ignore the fact that in one era in some social groups a co-residing grandmother may have been a revered and powerful patriarch, in another was housed only with extreme reluctance with everyone hoping that she would soon die, while in another she is viewed as an old friend who can claim the rights of friendship but no more, is to these scholars to miss the most essential changes which have occurred in familial systems over the past 500 years.
>
> (Anderson 1980: 35)

The lesson to be taken here is that figures rarely explain phenomena, indeed they may often mislead by disguising diversity. Frustratingly, however, the kinds of evidence we would require to confirm or refute the attitudes alluded to above are few and far between. Where information does exist, this has implications for the scale at which a study is pitched, for if we wish to investigate the detailed dynamics of relationships, such as those between generations in the same household, then we have to study sources at the micro-scale. This frequently means selecting samples which may be highly atypical. In such cases, one must balance the ability to generalize on the basis of random sampling – thus losing meaning – against the possibilities of understanding an issue in greater depth by deliberately selecting particular cases and thereby losing representativeness.

Case studies

The chapter discusses two very different examples based on primary and secondary archival research. However, in both matters of method and interpretation are central. In the first, social surveys conducted in England between the 1890s and 1940s are discussed with a view to discerning the social circumstances of older people in poverty. The second considers photographic images from 1850 to 1950, focusing upon fishing communities in Scotland and North East England to assess the range and character of representations of ageing and identity in selected archives.

Case study 1: Social surveys: family life and poverty in old age

A lively debate exists as to the relative importance and respective roles of family and state support for older people in the past. Yet while historians have explored a good deal of data for the nineteenth century and postwar investigators have examined and re-examined sample communities in some depth (Townsend 1957; Phillipson *et al.* 2000), the first half of the twentieth century is curiously deficient in research. In part this is because of the regulation preventing access to original census enumeration schedules until 100 years have elapsed.

In the period that saw the advent of old age pensions in 1908 and ended with the imposition of the retirement condition in 1948, the consideration of later life was heavily outweighed by the major issue of unemployment. The marginality of older people rendered them invisible from social commentary, and fieldwork into family budgets saw old age as largely peripheral to the nuclear family with children. Thus researching the experience of later life using data from social surveys involves making central issues that were not considered such at the time.

The process

While official surveys (e.g. Departmental Committee on Old-Age Pensions 1919) provide markers against which to contextualize the experience of interwar ageing, secondary analysis involves undertaking a comparative study of published community-level social surveys (Macnicol 1998: 265–84). Several projects, largely based on Rowntree's model for calculating family budgets and life-cycle poverty, were analysed. Among these were: Bowley's Five Towns surveys (Bowley and Burnett-Hurst 1915; Bowley and Hogg 1925); Caradog Jones's (1934) Merseyside study; Tout's (1938) Bristol and Ford's (1934) Southampton research, and Rowntree's (1941) restudy of York. However, as Gordon (1988a: 9) comments, 'in none of these do we get anything other than a most bare description of the kin composition of families', and it is only in the *New Survey of London* (1928–33) (Llewellyn Smith 1932) – a conscious attempt to rerun Booth's epic analysis of *The Life and Labour of the People in London* (1889–93) – that more detailed primary research into the composition and incomes of households containing older people is facilitated. The original Household Sample Cards now form a computerized dataset which may be consulted in the British Library of Political and Economic Science (see Appendix), or at the University of Essex. Over 28,000 working-class households containing some 98,400 people were surveyed, including several dozen East London pensioners who were interviewed concerning their living conditions, domestic budgets and attitudes towards various forms of support. Nevertheless, the survey excluded those living in institutions, thus eliminating some 6 per cent of all aged persons.

Findings

From Booth's pioneering empirical work on *The Aged Poor* (Booth 1894) to the Nuffield Report on *Old People* (Rowntree 1947), a series of pervasive 'expert' definitions is revealed in the classification of older people by social investigators. Since the 1830s, official statistics had lumped together the aged, the chronic sick and the temporarily disabled as 'non-able-bodied'. After 1890, however, statistics on outdoor relief teased apart these categories, while Booth's findings clarified the link between old age and want, showing between one-fifth and one-third of all persons over the age of 65 to be in poverty. His *Aged Poor* revealed, however, that this arbitrarily selected age was far from synonymous with the onset of senescence. Nevertheless, Rowntree's (1901) tabulations failed to distinguish between old age and other 'causes' of poverty, noting only 'incapacity of chief wage-earner through accident, illness or old age'. Each inquiry encountered difficulties in analysing intergenerational transfer incomes and other hidden forms of maintenance, and was forced to speculate from qualitative evidence given over in specimen case histories. Savings were almost impossible to discern and, clearly, such snapshot, cross-sectional surveys could not calculate the degree to which individuals had been able or inclined to put by for the hardships of later life at an earlier stage in the life course. Tout, meanwhile, found poverty to be 'characteristic of a family, not of an individual, who is said to be in poverty only because he happens to be a member of a family' (Tout 1938: 36). Considered in such terms, the growing numbers of old people living alone outside the family context received scant attention.

Budgetary calculations assumed that pensioners, despite (or because of) high fuel costs, ate less and required fewer clothes, the *New Survey* asserting that 'the condition of poverty varies inversely with the scale of income and directly with the scale of wants and both the scales of income and of wants tend to diminish with old age'. 'Clearly', it continued, 'the problem of the relation of old age to poverty is to a preponderant extent a women's problem, just as that of unemployment is mainly concerned with men' (Llewellyn Smith 1932: 190–1). Although older women outnumbered men in a ratio of 3:2, the focus was on the male breadwinner, while domestic, unpaid labour was scarcely considered. We have to wait until the postwar Nuffield surveys of Rowntree (1947) and Sheldon (1948) for the 'problem of age' to be fully attended to in social research.

Nonetheless, some of the complexity of attitudes towards older people is evident. The case reports collected in the field research for the *New Survey*, for example, reveal a moral language on the part of the interviewer not dissimilar to that used by Public Assistance Committee officials in its readiness to attribute measures of deservingness, self-help, cleanliness and providence:

> Miss S. seemed to be rather a grubby woman. Her clothes were very, very untidy, not very clean and not too well cared for. She said, however, that she always took care to go out looking neat, and that I must not judge her by her morning clothes as she had just got up . . . She said that she always buys a 1s 8d bottle of Guinness each week, as when you get old you must have nourishing things. I rather wondered whether she drinks . . . as there was a large bottle of beer on the table.
>
> (Llewellyn Smith 1932: 459)

This quotation also reveals a tension between meanings offered through the self-representations of individuals (Miss S.) and the definitions implied by institutional regulation (the influence of poor law morality on the interviewer). Investigations, such as that conducted by Mass-Observation (1948), provide considerable corroboration, albeit impressionistic.

Practical lessons

The minute level of detail provided set against the geographical unevenness of coverage (no rural samples, for instance) means that anything like a comprehensive overview is impossible. Complex patterns of assistance cannot be fully examined from the study of household structure since kin networks clearly stretched beyond individual households. This is especially true since Gordon's analysis of the *New Survey* reveals very little evidence of co-residence of older and younger relatives (Gordon 1988a: 46). However, lack of breadth is compensated for by the depth of insight provided concerning household relations, and, more particularly, the character of relationships via specimen case studies. These, at least, provide some indication of the degree and quality of assistance. Moreover, related work by social historians is rich in suggesting family and household strategies and may be usefully compared with oral accounts from contemporary pensioners who were children during the 1920s–1940s (Roberts 1984). One ought, nevertheless, to be wary about drawing broader conclusions about social attitudes towards later life on the basis of analysis that avowedly concentrates on the experiences of only the more impoverished members of society, even though that minority was a sizeable one.

Further research

Gordon's work on the *New Survey* suggests that the role of kin, both nuclear and extended, was slight and that older people were thus heavily reliant upon institutional mechanisms of support (Gordon 1988a, 1988b). While contributing to ongoing controversies (Thomson 1984; Hunt 1989), it also has clear implications for policy in the present. Our sample analysis lends some weight to the thesis while exploring the nature of relations between older claimants and the welfare system. While the findings require to be set within a wider framework for the examination of support that focuses upon the experience of work, retirement, families and poverty over the life course, the absence of longitudinal samples of personal incomes creates a major obstacle.

Funding sources

The present work began as part of an ESRC-funded project. Research of this nature remains relevant to the 'Growing Older' programme (see Appendix) and to the 'Lifecourse, Lifestyles and Health Thematic Priority' (Phillipson *et al.* 2000). Meanwhile, given its founder's own interests in the area, the Rowntree Foundation (see Appendix) could be a topical source. Depending upon how the questions are framed, the quantitative scale of a study such as the *New Survey* may be sufficient to justify the use of research assistance.

Case study 2: *Photographic images of age and generation*

Much of the history of old age deals with images and attitudes. Stereotypes are often visual, and pictures are especially important in constructing representations of later life (Blaikie and Hepworth 1997). The advent of photography in the late 1830s, its popularization as the nineteenth century progressed, and the subsequent development of photographic collections allows us to examine the construction of stereotypical images, to assess the extent of material available, to observe both the contexts within which images were created and to examine the ways in which they have sub-sequently been arranged and assessed. The following discussion summarizes a pilot study conducted across a range of British archives, looking at East Coast fishing communities in the period from 1850 to 1914.

The process

Initial contact was made with a number of national, regional and local holdings. In one case (Hulton Deutsch Collection, now Hulton Getty) fur-ther investigation was precluded by the organization's policy of not allow-ing public access to the archive, but instead charging a search fee following requests for specific photographs. However, in the remaining cases visits were arranged, access was granted, and I was able to interview curators concerning their collections. During this process I was informed of further sources of material and subsequently extended coverage to include these. The following archives thus provided the material on which the study was based: Scottish Ethnological Archive and Scottish Photographic Archive, Edinburgh; Newhaven Heritage Museum; Whitby Archives Heritage Centre and the Sutcliffe Gallery, Whitby; National Museum of Photography, Brad-ford; St Andrews University collections; the Scottish Fisheries Museum, Anstruther; Johnston Collection, Wick; the Orkney Library, Kirkwall; Shetland Museum, Lerwick; and George Washington Wilson Collection, University of Aberdeen.

The extent to which older people feature within the overall body of material in any one collection proved difficult to assess, since no one index included 'old age' as a separate category. However, most operated a system which enabled rapid access to relevant material: such headings as 'fishing: baiting lines' [an activity primarily reserved for elders], 'family and relations', or 'health and welfare' incorporated most images of older people or inter-generational portraits. While such classifications may accurately represent the key roles and relationships of older people during the period, curatorial biases in allocating images to pre-selected categories need also to be borne in mind. This is particularly so in the case of 'local characters', a classifica-tion operating in every collection and serving to create a series of iconic portraits of legendary local figures, eccentrics and ageing heroes (often captioned with copious narratives). Such individuals were clearly remark-able precisely because of their atypicality.

The size of even small collections meant that research had to be selective. In this, I opted either for in-depth scrutiny within particular index head-ings, or to consider the photographs taken by specific photographers. Thus it was possible to evaluate the ways in which particular categories were constructed.

Findings

Photographs are documents but this does not mean they are documentary in the factual sense. Visual images do not simply mirror reality; rather, they reflect the cultural beliefs and stylistic conventions of their time. Thus pictures of old age cannot be understood as renditions of an unchanging essence, but must be regarded as context-bound representations of popular ideals about how older people should appear. We are familiar with a wide range of stereotypes varying from grace, wisdom, and familial contentment to loneliness, mental senility and the physically grotesque. Nevertheless, particular historical periods emphasize differing characteristics. For example, in an earlier study several themes emerged from an analysis of Victorian paintings: these included older people being a focus on account of their longevity, facial features providing evidence of virtue or ancient married couples presenting an idyll of lifelong companionship, and scenes in which older people exemplified specific later-life roles, such as the comforting widow consoling her daughter whose husband is lost in an accident at sea (Blaikie and Hepworth 1997).

In like fashion, the present analysis of photographic material indicates a number of traits from which a typology, or iconography of old age might be constructed. First, many Victorian photographs imitate the artistic conventions of the period. Photographic pioneers Hill and Adamson acknowledged the influence of Vermeer in their depiction of multigenerational family groups in Newhaven, while the late nineteenth-century tradition of social realism is reflected in portrayals of elderly sailors as the maritime counterparts of the salt of the earth. George Washington Wilson's 'An Old Salt' is a definitive example, along with Sutcliffe's 'Retired from the Sea', both men bewhiskered and chewing on clay pipes.

Second, many images suggest stereotypical roles: older people as wise elders (Sutcliffe's 'Free Education', taken on the Fish Pier, Whitby, where a local fisherman is holding forth to a group of schoolchildren); generational continuity of occupational tasks (Washington Wilson's 'Three Generations of Newhaven Fishwives') or contented older couples, posed in black to indicate their retired status.

Such formality as appears in most portraits was enforced by contemporary camera technology, which required sitters to remain still for minutes at a time. Unfortunately, this means that little can be read into the comportment of older people by way of analysing their body language. Nevertheless, a third category concerns stereotypes of decrepitude. These range from an old man straining to hear a child by cupping his hand around his ear while resting his other hand atop a walking stick, to gnarled and bent figures standing emblematically before equally decayed old buildings (Blaikie 1994).

Fourth, there are the aforementioned 'local characters'. Several photo-graphers amassed images of 'personalities', hence, for instance, the sub-categories 'Kay personalities', 'Manson – personalities', 'personalities – Rattar', and so on, among the catalogue files of the Shetland Museum. As elsewhere, these include copious images of elderly neighbourhood eccentrics, often possessing bizarre nicknames, wearing outlandish garb, and afflicted by oddly shaped bodies or strange facial features.

Fifth – although less so in maritime communities than in the rural back-waters – there were images of older people taken because they represented the final bearers of vanishing skills or a way of life. This usage of photo-graphy as a means of archiving for posterity reflected a tendency to caricature seen in the classification of 'East Coast types', such as the 'The Scottish Fishwife' and 'The Deck-Chair Man' later depicted in railway advertising posters. It is, of course, the function of museums and other archives to collect and preserve images in this way. For our purposes, this requires an appreciation of the ways in which our 'heritage' acquires a romantic tinge as these aged survivors are invested with an aura of quaintness (Blaikie 1997). For example, the apparently authentic harmony of extended kin relationships in 'the past' suggested by many pictures has to be set against what we know from alternative historical readings.

Finally, and relatedly, many images must be regarded as ambiguous. An image such as Sutcliffe's 'Morning and Evening', which pictures an old man holding his nephew, could be read as symbolically representing a shared sense of the social marginality of childhood and old age (Hockey and James 1993: 18–21), yet it could equally plausibly be argued that both children and elders were significantly involved in preparatory tasks such as baiting lines and that this image celebrates the extended bonds of family in the economic well-being of fishing communities. Photographs are a par-ticularly malleable source, and much depends upon the cultural baggage the viewer brings to the process of interpretation (Blaikie 2001).

Practical lessons

Concentrating upon particular localities, distinguished by a common at-tachment to fishing, allows for a degree of community-level and individual biographical detail in contextualizing images. By the same token, findings have limited application and cannot be said to offer a representative cross-section of, say, attitudes towards older people in British history more gener-ally. Nevertheless, the approach adopted does generate questions that can be tested in other social settings. For example, the ways in which older people appear to have been selected because they represent scarce vestiges of dying trades and traditions could be compared with how they are repres-ented in farming or urban communities, as could their differing roles within family and community. However, images remain impressionistic, and analyses must be conducted in relation to other forms of evidence –

such as census material, oral history and Parliamentary papers, as well as postcards and cartoons – that corroborate or refute the photographic record (Blaikie and Macnicol 1986). Social constructionism points to the dangers of interpreting images from the vantage point of the present without recourse to such triangulation. As Thane (2000: 5–6) surmises,

> visual, cultural, definitions of old age at all times might conflict, and coexist, with both chronological and functional definitions. People might 'look old' but remain vigorous . . . Possibly more people 'looked old' in earlier centuries than were chronologically old by modern definitions, hence 'old people' may have been more visible in most communities than the demographic statistics suggest.

Further research

With the opportunities offered by computer technology, many local, national and international collections have now been scanned into electronic image banks that can be easily, if not always freely, accessed over the internet. However, the sheer volume of individual prints in each archive means that such electronic databases only include a limited range of images, with the added problem of bias in their selection. For smaller collections, there is still no substitute for travelling to the original archives. Photographs are just one of the visual media awaiting serious historical analysis by gerontologists (Blaikie 1994). If anything, paintings, postcards, cartoons and the moving image are even less researched, despite the relative ease of access to many collections, for example the Centre for the Study of Cartoons and Caricature, University of Kent (see Appendix). Portraits of older people may be found in almost any local or national art gallery.

Funding sources

The nature of the fieldwork lends itself to brief visits to archives dispersed across several locations. Thus travel expenses are a prime consideration. A budget is required both for obtaining copies of prints and permissions to reproduce selected images, but since the aim is to analyse material already organized into collections, no costs are involved in the compilation of databases. Because of a long association with art history, most picture research is considered within the remit of humanities rather than social science research. However, the Wellcome Trust has recognized the potential of visual archives for explorations in the social history of medicine. The Wellcome Trust Medical Photographic Library houses a collection of over 160,000 pictures as well as a Medical Film and Video Library (see Appendix). The above research was sponsored by a small grant from the Nuffield Foundation (see Appendix).

Conclusion

In questioning the master narrative of modernization, historians have emphasized the 'diversity of arrangements in past societies' (Troyansky 1997: 49). Both those who rely on quantitative sources – predominantly demographers and economic historians – and those who have analysed cultural representations in more distant times find ambiguity and ambivalence in attitudes and behaviour. Such scepticism, compared with earlier claims for rather less nuanced positions (e.g. Cowgill and Holmes 1972), reflects real refinement in methodology.

Before any source may be used, the researcher must ask questions of its provenance and subject the process by which the information came to be recorded to careful scrutiny. The sources considered here – social surveys and photographs – were collected for very different reasons and illustrate varying facets of the experience of ageing in the past. Nevertheless, they cannot stand alone: both must be subjected to a process of triangulation through comparison with the stories given by alternative sources; and neither may be regarded as conveying uncontestable truths.

It is possible, though rare, to integrate data through multiple source studies. For example, Smith has developed a micro-historical approach to derive pauper 'case histories' from nominal linkage between family reconstitution and Poor Law account books (Smith 1998). While such analyses can deliver significant results, they are extremely time-consuming given the very narrow, often single-parish level of coverage. In many instances, studies based on one time period will only provide information relevant to that era. However, rather than disregard such studies as overly specific, we might valuably attempt synthetic overview by developing a dialogue between varying approaches and time periods (Thane 2000: 3). Furthermore, the experiences of specific generations, cohorts and individuals can illuminate human behaviour under circumstances, such as war (Coleman 1997) or depression (Elder 1974), which are themselves repeatable. Such comparative analysis is critical to the development of long-run perspectives.

In an overview of postwar surveys, Thane illustrates the complexity of intergenerational relationships and transfers within families (Thane 1998). Although evidence for non-financial exchanges is limited and anecdotal, it being the duty of no one agency to record such, a major theme has been the emphasis upon reciprocity rather than the passivity of elders. Against this, our interpretation of the policy process is premised on particular perceptions of the life course (Kohli 1988). For the most part, the traces it leaves in its historical record reflect definitions that have emerged from the regulators of official knowledge rather than its subjects. However, ageing identities are constructed not simply through state regulation but according to how individuals negotiated their relationship to such impositions and external perceptions (Troyansky 1997: 56). For this reason, analysis should be aimed wherever possible at deconstructing official discourses while setting these against the rarer popular testimonies of older people themselves. Given the intractability of much information, the exercise provides a challenging test of the historian's craft, a skill that must pitch ingenuity on the one hand against circumspection on the other.

References

Achenbaum, W.A. and Stearns, P.N. (1978) Old age and modernization, *The Gerontologist*, 18: 307–12.

Anderson, M. (1980) *Approaches to the History of the Western Family, 1500–1914*. London: Macmillan.

Ariès, P. (1962) *Centuries of Childhood*. London: Jonathan Cape.

Blaikie, A. (1994) Photographic memory, ageing and the life course, *Ageing and Society*, 14(4): 479–97.

Blaikie, A. (1997) Beside the sea: visual imagery, ageing and heritage, *Ageing and Society*, 17(6): 629–48.

Blaikie, A. (1999) *Ageing and Popular Culture*. Cambridge: Cambridge University Press.

Blaikie, A. (2001) Photographs in the cultural account: contested narratives and collective memory in the Scottish islands, *Sociological Review*, 49(3): 345–67.

Blaikie, A. and Hepworth, M. (1997) Representations of old age in painting and photography, in A. Jamieson, S. Harper and C. Victor (eds) *Critical Approaches to Ageing and Later Life*, pp. 102–17. Buckingham: Open University Press.

Blaikie, A. and Macnicol, J. (1986) Towards an anatomy of ageism: society, social policy and the elderly between the wars, in C. Phillipson, M. Bernard and P. Strang (eds), *Dependency and Interdependency in Old Age: Theoretical Perspectives and Policy Alternatives*, pp. 95–104. Beckenham: Croom Helm.

Booth, C. (1889–1903) *Life and Labour of the People in London*, 17 vols. London: Macmillan.

Booth, C. (1894) *The Aged Poor in England and Wales*. London: Macmillan.

Bowley, A.L. and Burnett-Hurst, A.R. (1915) *Livelihood and Poverty*. London: Bell.

Bowley, A.L. and Hogg, M.H. (1925) *Has Poverty Diminished?* London: King.

Caradog Jones, D. (1934) *The Social Survey of Merseyside*, 3 vols. Liverpool: Liverpool University Press.

Coleman, P. (1997) Last scene of all, *Generations Review*, 7(1): 2–5.

Cowgill, D.O. and Holmes, L. (eds) (1972) *Aging and Modernization*. New York, NY: Appleton-Century-Crofts.

Departmental Committee on Old Age Pensions, *Parliamentary Papers* (1919), Cmd. 411, Vol. 27, Appendix, Minutes of Evidence.

Elder, G.H. (1974) *Children of the Great Depression*. Chicago, IL: University of Chicago Press.

Finley, M. (1984) The elderly in classical antiquity, *Ageing and Society*, 4(4): 391–408.

Ford, P. (1934) *Work and Wealth in a Modern Port*. London: Allen & Unwin.

Gordon, C. (1988a) *The Myth of Family Care? The Elderly in the Early 1930s*, STICERD (Suntory Toyota International Centre for Economics and Related Disciplines) *Welfare State Programme Discussion Paper* no. 29. London: London School of Economics.

Gordon, C. (1988b) Familial support for the elderly in the past: the case of London's working class in the early 1930s, *Ageing and Society*, 8(3): 287–320.

Hannah, L. (1986) *Inventing Retirement: The Development of Occupational Pensions in Britain*. Cambridge: Cambridge University Press.

Hindess, B. (1973) *The Use of Official Statistics in Sociology*. London: Macmillan.

Hockey, J. and James, A. (1993) *Growing Up and Growing Old: Ageing and Dependency in the Life Course*. London: Sage Publications.

Hunt, E.H. (1989) Paupers and pensioners: past and present, *Ageing and Society*, 9(4): 407–30.

Johnson, P. (1985) *The Economics of Old Age in Britain: A Long-run View, 1881–1981*, CEPR Discussion Paper no. 47. London: Centre for Economic Policy Research.

Johnson, P. and Thane, P. (eds) (1998) *Old Age from Antiquity to Post-modernity*. London: Routledge.

Johnson, P., Conrad, C. and Thomson, D. (eds) (1989) *Workers versus Pensioners: Intergenerational Justice in an Ageing World*. Manchester: CEPR/Manchester University Press.

Kohli, M. (1988) Ageing as a challenge for sociological theory, *Ageing and Society*, 8(3): 367–94.

Laslett, P. (1976) The wrong way through the telescope: a note on literary evidence in sociology and in historical sociology, *British Journal of Sociology*, 27(3): 319–42.

Laslett, P. (1977) The history of aging and the aged, in P. Laslett, *Family Life and Illicit Love in Earlier Generations*, pp. 174–213. Cambridge: Cambridge University Press.

Laslett, P. (1989) *A Fresh Map of Life: The Emergence of the Third Age*. London: Weidenfeld and Nicolson.

Llewellyn Smith, H. (1932) *The New Survey of London Life and Labour*, 10 vols. London: King.

Macnicol, J. (1998) *The Politics of Retirement in Britain, 1878–1948*. Cambridge: Cambridge University Press.

Mass-Observation (1948) Old age, *Bulletin*, New Series, No. 21.

Minois, G. (1989) *History of Old Age: From Antiquity to the Renaissance*. Cambridge: Polity Press.

National Galleries of Scotland (2001) *Rembrandt's Women* (exhibition notes).

Parkin, T.G. (1998) Ageing in antiquity: status and participation, in P. Johnson and P. Thane (eds) *Old Age from Antiquity to Post-modernity*, pp. 19–42. London: Routledge.

Pelling, M., and Smith, R.M. (eds) (1991) *Life, Death, and the Elderly: Historical Perspectives*. London: Routledge.

Phillipson, C., Bernard, M., Phillips, J. and Ogg, J. (2000) *The Family and Community Life of Older People*. London: Routledge.

Roberts, E. (1984) *A Woman's Place: An Oral History of Working-class Women, 1980–1940*. Oxford: Basil Blackwell.

Rowntree, B.S. (1901) *Poverty: A Study of Town Life*. London: Nelson.

Rowntree, B.S. (1941) *Poverty and Progress: A Second Social Survey of York*. London: Longman.

Rowntree, B.S. (1947) *Old People: Report of a Survey Committee on the Problems of Ageing and the Care of Old People*. London: The Nuffield Foundation/Oxford University Press.

Shakespeare, W. (1906) *Shakespeare: Complete Works*, ed. W.J. Craig. Oxford: Oxford University Press.

Shegog, R.F.A. (ed.) (1981) *The Impending Crisis of Old Age*. Oxford: Nuffield Provincial Hospitals Trust/Oxford University Press.

Sheldon, J.H. (1948) *The Social Medicine of Old Age*. London: The Nuffield Foundation/Oxford University Press.

Smith, R.M. (1984) The structured dependence of the elderly as a recent development: some sceptical historical thoughts, *Ageing and Society*, 4(4): 409–28.

Smith, R.M. (1998) Ageing and well-being in early modern England: pension trends and gender preferences under the English Old Poor Law *c.* 1650–1800, in P. Johnson and P. Thane (eds) *Old Age from Antiquity to Post-modernity*, pp. 64–95. London: Routledge.

Thane, P. (1995) The cultural history of old age, *Australian Cultural History*, 14: 23–39.

Thane, P. (1998) The family lives of old people, in P. Johnson and P. Thane (eds) *Old Age from Antiquity to Post-modernity*, pp. 180–210. London: Routledge.

Thane, P. (2000) *Old Age in English History*. Oxford: Oxford University Press.

Thomas, K. (1977) Age and authority in early modern England, *Proceedings of the British Academy*, LXII: 205–48.

Thomson, D. (1984) The decline of social welfare: falling state support for the elderly since early Victorian times, *Ageing and Society*, 4(4): 451–82.

Tout, H. (1938) *The Standard of Living in Bristol*. Bristol: Arrowsmith.

Townsend, P. (1957) *The Family Life of Old People: An Inquiry in East London*. London: Routledge and Kegan Paul.

Townsend, P. (1981) The structured dependency of the elderly: a creation of social policy in the twentieth century, *Ageing and Society*, 1(1): 5–28.

Troyansky, D. (1997) Historical research into ageing, old age and older people, in A. Jamieson, S. Harper and C. Victor (eds) *Critical Approaches to Ageing and Later Life*, pp. 49–62. Buckingham: Open University Press.

Wall, R. (1984) Residential isolation of the elderly: a comparison over time, *Ageing and Society*, 4(4): 483–503.

Wilson, A. (1980) The infancy of the history of childhood: an appraisal of Philippe Ariès, *History and Theory*, 19(2): 133–53.

4

Using existing research and statistical data: secondary data analysis

Christina Victor

Introduction

In Britain there are a wide variety of existing data sources available to the social gerontologist. We are a 'data rich' country. Other chapters in this book consider the issues involved in undertaking primary research using historical, contemporary and 'cultural' data sources. In this chapter we concentrate upon routinely available statistical data, as this is the most common form of 'secondary' analysis and is the most readily available source of data, especially for the 'student' researcher. Furthermore the emphasis is primarily upon government-sponsored data sets (see Hakim 1982 for a comprehensive if dated resumé of major datasets). However, many of the issues raised apply equally to the reanalysis of historical and other more documentary or archive material and to the (re)use of more locally based empirical material.

What is secondary data analysis?

For either pragmatic or resource reasons gerontological researchers in the UK (and elsewhere) may choose to answer their research question via the exploitation of existing data sets (rather than collecting original data). This is conventionally termed 'secondary data analysis' and is an approach that is common within the UK social science community. Secondary analysis may be defined, according to Arber (2001) as 'the (re)analysis and

Table 4.1   Trends in self-reported long-standing limiting illness 1972–98

	Age			
	65–74		75+	
	M	F	M	F
1972	36	39	46	49
1975	37	38	45	54
1979	35	41	44	56
1981	40	45	53	54
1985	38	38	43	51
1989	37	36	44	53
1991	40	34	46	51
1993	41	39	45	52
1995	37	37	41	52
1996	42	40	50	53
1998	36	39	48	51

Source: Bridgwood *et al.* 2000: Table 7.1

interpretation of existing data initially collected for another purpose by another researcher or organisation'. This broad definition is largely uncontested and is largely accepted throughout Europe, Australasia and North America. Within this very broad definition we can identify two different approaches to the goal of 'reanalysis and interpretation' of existing data. The first approach involves examination and rescrutiny of the published data sets such as, for example, examining trends in the prevalence of long-standing limiting illness (see Table 4.1), the characteristics of older people (Mathieson and Summerfield 1999), particular subgroups of the population or trends in the health of the population as measured by mortality data (Charlton and Murphy 1997). This approach simply involves the collation and scrutiny of data published as tables or graphs within a range of existing publications. Many of these data/tables are available via the Office for National Statistics (ONS) website or other government/academic websites listed in Appendix. In contrast the second approach involves obtaining the original data and reconsidering and reanalysing this to undertake new analyses, interpretations or answer novel research questions. This type of approach may require a greater degree of statistical expertise than the former approach. Regardless of the approach adopted the emphasis here is upon using existing data to develop new insights, address theoretical or conceptual issues, or try to answer questions which the data set was never intended or designed to answer! Originality in research is not solely about the collection of new or novel data sets. Rather it is novelty of the research question and the new insights generated that defines originality in research, not necessarily the novelty of the data set.

Secondary data analysis is not an activity unique to gerontologists. Rather it is an approach often used by social scientists interested in a whole range of different areas. Neither is secondary data analysis particularly new. Ever since written records have been kept researchers have been interrogating such sources to answer specific questions, as the chapter by Blaikie illustrates.

What types of data can be used for secondary analysis?

Secondary data analysis is an 'umbrella' term that covers a wide variety of different types of research question, data sets and data sources. While there is often a focus upon the reuse of statistical data sets, as exemplified by the work of Arber and Ginn (1991), there are many other sources of data including qualitative material, and letters, books or diaries can form the basis for this type of analysis. This aspect of secondary analysis is perhaps best exemplified by the Mass-Observation Archive at the University of Sussex and discussed in this book in the chapter by Sheridan. Secondary analysis and the use of existing data sources is a very flexible research approach and one particularly suited to the student researcher who is unlikely to have the resources to undertake extensive original data collection. Such data sources can provide the empirical material for undergraduate/ postgraduate degree dissertations.

The overwhelming majority of gerontological 'secondary analysis' in the UK is based upon the re-examination of existing statistical data. Again, the overwhelming majority of the data subject to reinterpretation and analysis is sponsored via the government and collected and managed via ONS. Such statistical data has a variety of different origins and is collected for a variety of different purposes. However, in undertaking secondary analysis users need a degree of awareness as to the original purpose of the survey as this inevitably circumscribes the remit, design and outcome of the data collection exercise. We may classify government-sponsored data into three broad categories:

- registration data;
- administrative data; and
- social profile/policy monitoring data.

For full details of all statistical material produced by the government see the Guide to Official Statistics published annually and available on the ONS website (see Appendix).

Registration data

Registration data relates to information derived from aspects of compulsory civil registration, i.e. births, marriages and deaths, introduced in the early nineteenth century. Each of these events is registered with the civil authorities at the district Registrar's Office. From individual acts such as the registration of the birth of a child or death of a citizen data are collated about the number of births, deaths and marriages taking place annually. From such data we can examine trends in family formation, changes in fertility and patterns of mortality. Such information is at the heart of information demonstrating the remarkable decreases in mortality and increases in life expectancy characteristic of the twentieth century. Full details of the availability of civil registration data are provided on the ONS website.

Census data

While not required for purposes of civil registration the decennial census is another 'compulsory' data collection exercise sponsored by the government. The census has taken place every 10 years since 1801 and provides the cornerstone for information concerning the demographic structure of the populations and a myriad of other social information. It also provides the information which enables us to combine data about births or deaths with the appropriate population denominators so that we can calculate rates, such as infant mortality or death rates, and then examine temporal or spatial trends. A vast amount of census data is available for secondary analysis and full details are available on the census website (see Appendix).

Administrative data

Administrative data are concerned with information collected as a result of the running and monitoring of specific services. This type of information is collected in areas such as health, housing and social care. However the information is collected for the purpose of, for example, examining the functioning of the NHS, as in the collection of data concerning 'waiting times' for operations or for monitoring specific areas of interest such as notifications of specific infectious diseases such as salmonella, and not primarily as research tools. However, the aspects of the social welfare system of interest to policy makers are not always those most relevant to the secondary analyist. Furthermore, the units used to collect the data also reflect the interests of policy makers and administrators. Hospital in-patient data is collected not by patient but by 'completed consultant episodes' (the period of care under the charge of a specific consultant). A single patient, during one spell in hospital, may experience periods of care under several different consultants and hence will appear as two (or more) completed consultant episodes. Nursing home data is presented in terms of beds rather than people or places. Hence the users of secondary analysis need to be mindful of the varying denominators used in the presentation of administrative data.

Social profile data

Social profile and monitoring data is a more eclectic and generic category that includes many of the major continuous national 'social' surveys such as the General Household Survey, the Labour Force Survey, the Family Expenditure Survey, the Family Resources Survey and the Health Survey for England. These social 'monitoring' surveys are usually undertaken annually. In addition various 'ad hoc' surveys are undertaken in response to specific policy questions such as the surveys of psychiatric morbidity or disability. Full details of the contents of such surveys are available from the ONS website. However, such surveys are rarely exclusively devoted to topics of later life, older people or ageing, although any representative general population survey will include substantial numbers of older people as the population aged 60+ constitutes approximately 20 per cent of the population. So a survey of 10,000 adults will contain, at best, 2000 people aged 60 and over and as few as 100 aged 85+. This makes analysis of specific subgroups of the older population, such as married women aged 85 or older, very problematic.

In addition not all surveys available for secondary use are government-sponsored as the series of British Social Attitudes Survey reports demonstrates. However, it is usually only the large data sets or those funded by agencies such as the Medical Research Council (MRC), Wellcome or Economic and Social Research Council (ESRC) that are deposited with the national data archive service. The ESRC 'Growing Older' (GO) programme should provide a rich source of data for secondary analysis as all data sets from the projects will eventually be deposited at the ESRC Data Archive. Secondary data is often, but not inevitably, held in archives (either electronic or paper) or libraries and as such may provide a comprehensive source of data on a particular subject (often in a single location). In a library we can examine the published reports of the General Household Survey reports that have been published since 1971. The most recent report published in 2001 is available online. In addition we can often obtain the 'raw' data sets in electronic form from archives such as the UK Data Archive at Essex University, including the Qualidata Archive. The Data Archive holds large-scale data sets collected for the government by ONS and others. It is not appropriate to list all the data sets held by the Archive as they are extensive (this is available from their website: see Appendix). The Data Archive also has links to the major United States and other national/international data archives. However, some indication of the range of material held is appropriate. The Archive holds large regular social surveys such as the General Household Survey and the Health Survey for England as well as 'ad hoc' surveys such as the Survey of Psychiatric Morbidity. Large-scale surveys including the British Social Attitudes and the British Crime Survey are also available. Most of these surveys are cross-sectional in nature but there are some longitudinal data available. Perhaps the best known are the National Child Development Studies (NCDS) and the 1970 Birth Cohort Study (BCS70) which have followed up at intervals all births in a specific week in 1958 and 1970 respectively. Wadsworth, in his chapter, makes imaginative use of material from the National Survey of Health and Development, a follow-up of the 1946 birth cohort, to illustrate the key methodological issues associated with longitudinal research and demonstrate the insights such data can shed upon the experience of ageing. More recently the British Household Panel Survey (BHPS), an annual survey of 5000 households, was established in 1991. Locally based data sets are also deposited at the Data Archive (although this policy is being abandoned to concentrate upon major holdings), such as the data collected by Wenger in North Wales. The Qualidata Archive holds qualitative material and also 'historical' survey data such as that collected by Townsend (1957) for his study of older people in the East End of London. Full details of holdings and the level of support provided are available from the UK Data Archive website and data are provided free to academic users.

The advantages of secondary data analysis

Secondary data analysis is concerned with the utilization of existing data sets to answer questions which the data were never intended to answer. Given this inherent limitation what are the attractions of reusing existing data? We can identify four basic advantages of using existing data: comprehensiveness, uniqueness, quality and value for money.

Secondary data analysis often offers researchers unique access to particular types of data, either in terms of the novelty of the methodology, the topic of the study, the inclusion of specific population subgroups, or the time span covered by the material. It is therefore often more comprehensive than locally commissioned studies. Often researchers are interested in specific population subgroups such as ethnic minority elders or older people living with their children, or the 'women in the middle'. It is extremely difficult to identify such groups and then to include them within a particular research project. One way to overcome this is to use existing data and combine data from different years of a particular survey, such as the General Household Survey (GHS), to generate sufficient numbers in the category of interest. This was the approach used by Evandrou (2000) to consider the health of ethnic minority elders. As mentioned previously, the availability of secondary data over a historical period enables the researcher to examine trends over time, provided that the data have been collected and documented using a consistent protocol. Examination of data concerning long-term limiting illness may, for example, offer some insight into the veracity (or otherwise) of the compression of morbidity hypothesis (see Table 4.1).

Many of the large-scale surveys available for secondary analysis have been conducted by the ONS or other highly reputable agencies such as the former Social and Community Planning Research (now the National Centre for Survey Research at City University), or sponsored by organizations such as the MRC. As such, considerable time and effort has been expended to ensure that the data collected are robust and of high quality. However, while much of the data produced by these types of surveys is of high quality, it should not be treated uncritically. From the researcher's perspective, however, secondary analysis offers a potentially large, rich and fairly robust source of data at comparatively little expense. Hence, for many researchers, secondary analysis offers considerable opportunities at least to investigate difficult or challenging research topics where it may be difficult for the researcher to gain access to the group (such as minority community members) or raise sensitive topics with research participants (such as sexual behaviour and lifestyle). It also offers the opportunity to test out ideas and develop new methodologies in advance of primary data collection.

The limitations of secondary data analysis

Secondary data analysis is not without its difficulties, and the majority of these stem from the conceptual basis of this type of analysis. The idealized model of social gerontological research is that in which researchers start off with a specific question (or hypothesis) they wish to investigate and design a research instrument to investigate this which includes 'operationalized' measures of the concepts under consideration. To investigate the extent of loneliness among older people the researchers might construct a questionnaire, which includes several questions designed to measure the concept of loneliness. However, in secondary analysis researchers always have to work with data that has been precollected without necessarily including adequate measures of interest to the researchers. Hence in using secondary analysis researchers have to look very closely at the concepts they wish to investigate and the measures included within the potential data set. For example, the theory of disengagement has been a prominent one in gerontological research. To examine the veracity of this theory requires some operationalized measures of 'disengagement'. Examination of, for example, the GHS may offer only proxy or indirect measures of disengagement in as much as this provides information about individuals who do (and do not) engage in a variety of leisure activities or social interaction. Hence such measures can only ever offer a partial or limited measurement of the concept of disengagement.

In addition to the issues concerning the overall content of government surveys there are also issues concerning the accuracy of measurement and recording of the data. Where the variables being measured appear, at first sight, to be hard and unambiguous there is still the potential for error. Mortality data would seem to be one of the most reliable and valid sources of data available to the secondary analyst. In Britain, where death certification is a legal requirement, we probably have a complete record of all deaths. However, the accuracy of other information provided on the death certificate may be subject to error. The most problematic aspect of certification is establishing cause of death, especially in the case of older people. Death certification is a task often undertaken by junior doctors under minimal supervision (Bloor 1991). Hence the accuracy of certification of cause of death cannot be taken for granted. Yet it is upon the diagnostic decisions of considerable numbers of individual doctors that data upon cause of death are collated. We may speculate that data derived from administrative records such as the waiting list information may be less than 100 per cent accurate and complete. Notification data for infectious diseases and cancer registrations demonstrate considerably less than 100 per cent completeness. Hence, while secondary data often derives from very reputable and credible sources, the researcher must always critically evaluate the completeness, accuracy, reliability and validity of the sources used.

Clearly the content of many of these surveys and routine data sources are constrained by matters of social and political policy. Many routine surveys are heavily policy influenced, hence reflect current concerns of policy makers. For example the Health Survey for England is designed to monitor progress towards key national health targets and *not* to monitor the health status of older people or examine inequalities in health. The political context, as well as the current state of knowledge and the nature of the predominant theoretical paradigm, can also influence both the initiation of specific surveys and their contents. Questions in the GHS concerned with share ownership and the availability of private medical insurance reflect the interests of the then Conservative administration in promoting both of these activities. Furthermore the assumptions and preconceptions of the survey sponsors or policy makers may further limit the content of such surveys (although a similar observation could be made about much 'original' research). The widespread acceptance by policy makers and government of the 'apocalyptic' demographic future based upon increasing numbers of (frail) older people combined with smaller and fragmented families stimulated research into the extent of informal care via the GHS. However, the definition of caring used was highly instrumental and task-orientated, as this was an attempt to try to estimate the potential problems that some future state would have to respond to if there were a decline in the availability of family carers as a result of changes in fertility and marriage patterns. Older people were conceptualized as passive recipients of care and the questions asked them who helped them with various tasks and not what help they provided to others. This illustrates the challenge for all researchers using this approach of exploiting existing data to answer novel questions or test specific theories within the constraints imposed by the original data collection methodology.

In addition, as many surveys are concerned with general population, there are often issues of sample size for those interested in studying old age or later life (or indeed any other population subgroup). Although the GHS has a total sample of approximately 10,000 households (20,000 people in 1998), this includes only 3234 people aged 65+, the majority of whom are aged 65–74. The GHS includes only about 1300 people aged 75+. Hence, in order to derive a meaningful sample of the 'oldest old' it would be necessary to combine data from several years. Also, general surveys such as GHS exclude 'institutional' population, so they are of limited utility for making generalizations about the total population of older people. Estimates of the prevalence of disability and chronic health problems among older people, based solely upon the GHS, significantly underestimate the 'true' extent of these problems within the population because of the exclusion of those 'in care'.

Furthermore, there is often a time lag between the collection of the data and the publication/availability of the data and results. Often this is in the order of two years, as data are not usually released until the relevant report has been published. However, this is not necessarily a major limitation, as few gerontological research questions are rendered irrelevant because of delay in the availability of data.

What types of questions can secondary data analysis investigate?

We can identify three major types of research in British gerontology, although of course a single study may address more than one type of research question. A similar typology of work can be applied to the investigations of gerontologists in other countries, although the balance between them will inevitably be different. These are empirical research, applied research and theoretical research. Empirical research is primarily concerned with generating knowledge about the world of older people and the nature and characteristics of this subset of the population. Much British gerontological work has been conducted within this paradigm and has sought to challenge many of the myths and stereotypes that abound concerning the nature of later life. Theoretical research is concerned with the development of theoretical insights or the testing of theoretically informed research questions. This is a much less well established branch of gerontology in the UK. Applied research has been a particular strength of British researchers. This type of research focuses upon questions of policy and practice at a local, regional, national (and perhaps international) level. Secondary data analysis can be used, in theory at least, to examine questions in each of these three different aspects of gerontological research. However, there is usually a focus upon the first type of approach. Furthermore, secondary analysis can be used to develop and suggest potential areas for research. For example, data on mortality from the World Health Organization (WHO) data set reveal that life expectancy in Britain is eight years less than that of France. As such this simple observation can be used to generate research questions as to what it is about the social fabric of France that results in this apparent mortality advantage. Secondary analysis can contribute both to the under-standing of the life course and later life and to generate new questions.

Another and overlying distinction in gerontological research can be made. This is the distinction between researching later life and the nature and characteristics of older people and the study of ageing. Given the paucity of longitudinal data sets in Britain it is this former aspect that has been stud-ied using secondary data analysis. However, some secondary analysis of longitudinal data is possible. For example, Pendry *et al.* (1999) have added to our knowledge about the dynamics of household change in later life by reanalysis of the Health and Lifestyle Survey and its seven-year follow-up. Clearly the British Household Panel Survey offers the potential for longitu-dinal secondary analysis. This may be an aspect of secondary analysis that will become more common with increased availability of longitudinal/panel data.

Case studies/examples

Several cases are presented in the following examples in order to illustrate differing approaches to secondary analysis in gerontological research. These case studies illustrate different types of points concerning strengths/weaknesses of using existing data. They also illustrate the range of different types of questions that may be investigated using various sources of readily available secondary data. However, it is important to note that such data are often collected to answer policy questions but researchers want to use them to answer theoretical/methodological/empirical questions, and this is always problematic.

Reinterpretation and analysis of published material

Perhaps the most accessible form of secondary analysis is the reuse and reanalysis of material already published in reports and books. This can be used to examine, for example, trends over time. A comparison of patterns of mortality by age in 1841 and 1999 demonstrates the very profound change in the epidemiology of death (Table 4.2). In 1841 a third of all deaths were accounted for by children compared with 1 per cent in 1999. Conversely, 75 per cent of deaths in 1999 were accounted for by people

Table 4.2   Percentage deaths by age: England and Wales 1841–1999

	% deaths	
	1841	*1999*
Infancy/childhood (0–14)	37	1.2
Young adults (15–34)	25	1.6
Mid life (35–64)	33	22.3
Later life	15	75.1

Source: Derived from OPCS 1992: Table 3 and Population Trends 2000: Table 6.1

aged 65+ compared with 15 per cent in 1841. Such simple analysis is fairly straightforward in that the record of deaths is probably complete. Although there may be some doubts about the accuracy of the age information for the 1841 data this is unlikely to change grossly the pattern displayed.

A more sophisticated and novel type of secondary analysis is when it is combined with the collection and analysis of original data. One question of interest to the gerontologist concerns the comparison of the experience of later life for the current cohort of elders with that of older people in the past. The availability of historical material offers the opportunity for the generation of some insight into this question. Examples of the use of the re-examination of historical data and its comparison with contemporary material is provided by Phillipson *et al.* (2001) and Victor *et al.* (2001). The latter study examined the comparison of the prevalence and patterns of loneliness among older people now with their postwar cohort by reusing the material gathered by Townsend (1957), Tunstall (1966) and Sheldon (1948). The purpose of the study was to consider if loneliness is more prevalent among current generations of elders compared with those experiencing old age in the immediate postwar era. This is an example of 'historical' gerontology – ways of looking at trends over time in the absence of any longitudinal or panel data. Clearly, for the material to be directly comparable we need to ensure that it was gathered in the same way using the same questions. These conditions are rarely fulfilled, for surveys are often modified over time. In this example there were four major areas of difference:

- variations in composition of samples;
- variations in question wording and how the concept of loneliness is operationalized;
- secular changes in the distribution of 'risk factors' for loneliness; and
- limitation of detailed analysis to material published in books.

While the wording of the questions was comparable, the major characteristics of the samples studied, in terms of age structure and percentage

Table 4.3   The prevalence of loneliness (%)

Domain	Sheldon	Townsend	Tunstall	ESRC
Often lonely	7.9	5.0	8.6	9.3
Sometimes lonely	13.3	22	25.2	37.1
Never lonely	78.8	72	66.1	53.6

Source: Victor *et al.* 2001

living alone, changed greatly over the intervening four decades. However, despite these secular changes the overall distribution of loneliness is reasonably similar between the studies (Table 4.3).

The Health Survey for England provides extensive clinical and prescribing information. Shah and Cook (2001) undertook secondary analysis of this data set to look at class-based inequalities among older people in the detection and treatment of hypertension. This was an attempt by the authors to analyse empirical national data to consider two current health policy concerns. These were the continuation into later life of class-based differences in health service use (the inverse care law of Tudor-Hart states that access to care is inversely related to social class – those from 'lower' social classes are less likely to receive care than the more privileged) and the concept of ageism in medicine (restricting access to care by older people or providing them with 'worse' quality care). The work of Shah and Cook (2001) neatly illustrates several of the conceptual difficulties experienced when using secondary analysis. To create a study of adequate power involved aggregation of data from 1992 to 1996 to generate a sufficiently large sample size, as the event of interest, hypertension, is comparatively rare even among those 65+. Key challenges were

- definition of hypertension;
- classification of adequacy of treatment; and
- classifying population into 'social class' bands.

This study found no evidence of either ageism or the operation of the inverse care law, as there was no obvious class gradient in either the detection or treatment of hypertension.

Developing novel methodologies using secondary analysis

Secondary analysis has contributed much to our understanding of later life. The work by Evandrou (2000) on minority health, Arber and Ginn (1991) and Falkingham and Victor (1991) looking at financial provision are just a selection of the examples of the use of secondary analysis in gerontology. Secondary analysis has been developed further by the work of Evandrou and Falkingham (2000). They have constructed what they term

Table 4.4   Example of pseudo-cohort data for England and Wales

Birth cohort	% women remaining childless	
	At age 30	At age 40
1920	30	20
1931	21	14
1946	15	10
1964	40	22*

Note: *'Projected' as the 1964 birth cohort, are not yet 40.
Source: Victor *et al.* 2001

'pseudo-cohorts' (or synthetic cohorts) for the analysis of trends in ageing and the likely future shape of the experience of old age. This study used GHS and other data to construct 'pseudo-cohorts' examining three sets of parameters: living arrangements, health, and access to resources. Using GHS data they constructed four 'pseudo' cohorts: those born in 1916–20, 1931–5, 1946–50 and 1961–5. These cohorts can then be tracked using GHS and other routine data. For example the 1916–20 group were 55–9 at the time of the 1975 GHS, 65–9 in the 1985 GHS and 75–9 at the 1995 GHS. While we cannot track the changes of individual group members we can track the progress of the group overall. In this form of analysis the unit examined is the cohort (or group) and data are expressed as group means or averages. Using the construction of group averages (e.g. the percentage living alone for each cohort, or the prevalence of chronic illness at specific ages) we can then compare differences between groups and consider how this may affect the likely experience of old age in the future. Table 4.4 compares patterns of childlessness at different ages between the four cohorts. This illustrates that, while 15 per cent of those in the 1950 cohort were childless at age 30, for those in the 1960 cohort it was 40 per cent.

This is clearly a very novel and useful development of the secondary analysis perspective. However it clearly only provides a partial insight into the variations in experiences between cohorts. Clearly the analysis, and therefore the questions that can be asked, is limited by the remit of the 'source surveys'. Hence it is fairly easy to examine trends in solo living but much less easy to track changes in the coresidence of parent and adult children as the relationships between household members are not always specified. Furthermore, the use of group averages to present the data means that variations within cohorts is unexamined. We may speculate that there is as much variation within cohorts as between them. Despite the conceptual limitations, this presents a useful example of how the analysis of existing data can be approached in a novel and informative fashion to facilitate the development of new insights into the current experience of old age/ageing and how this may change for future generations. This serves to remind us of the importance of distinguishing 'true' ageing effects from period or cohort effects (see the chapters by Jamieson and Wadsworth) and serves to emphasize how much the social context influences the ageing experience.

Ethical issues

It is too often assumed that, because there are no respondents or research participants, ethical issues do not impinge upon secondary analysis. However, there are, of course, ethical issues to be considered in secondary analysis. Like other aspects of research secondary analysis also involves the issue of consent. Except when using published data and in other rare situations, secondary analysis usually requires the consent of the original organization that collected the data and/or the archive where it is stored. This is usually granted as part of the process of gaining access to the data and remains an important consideration. Those who deposit data in archives or make it available for secondary research usually require acknowledgement in any resultant publications or dissertations. This is an aspect of 'research etiquette' that should not be ignored and secondary data should not be passed off as one's own – that is plagiarism or theft!

Conclusion

In Britain, and many other countries especially Europe, North America and Australasia, there is a wealth of material available for reuse by the research community. The advantages of using existing data relate to the availability of such data, its comprehensiveness and the potential it offers to undertake investigations of interrelations such as class inequalities in health or the analysis of specific groups (Evandrou 2000), relationships and subgroup analysis. The major problems centre upon the constraints imposed by the reliance upon the initial set of questions asked, e.g. HSE (Health Survey for England) does not ask income questions, and the initial focus of study (often policy-related). However, this is often a very good approach for students and sole researchers, as this type of study does not require much in the way of financial resources, although the time involved can be considerable. The enduring challenge of secondary analysis for the gerontologist is to be able to use existing data sets to pose (and answer) innovative and informative questions about old age and later life.

References

Arber, S. (2001) Secondary analysis of survey data, in N. Gilbert (ed.) *Researching Social Life*, 2nd edition. London: Sage Publications.

Arber, S. and Ginn, J. (1991) *Gender and Later Life*. London: Sage Publications.

Bloor, M. (1991) A minor offence: the variable and socially constructed character of death certification in a Scottish city, *Journal of Health and Social Behaviour*, 32: 273–87.

Bridgwood, A., Lily, R., Thomas, M. *et al.* (2000) *Living in Britain: Results from the 1998 GHS*. London: Office for National Statistics.

Charlton, J. and Murphy, M. (eds) (1997) *The Health of Adult Britain*. London: HMSO.

Evandrou, M. (2000) Ethnic inequalities in health, *Health Statistics Quarterly*, 8: 20–8.

Evandrou, M. and Falkingham, J. (2000) Looking back to look forward: lessons from four birth cohorts for ageing in the twenty-first century, *Population Trends*, 99: 27–36.

Falkingham, J. and Victor, C.R. (1991) The myth of the woopie, *Ageing and Society*, 11(4): 471–93.

Hakim, C. (1982) *Secondary Data Analysis in Social Research*. London: Allen & Unwin.

Mathieson, J. and Summerfield, C. (1999) *Social Focus on Older People*. London: Office for National Statistics.

Pendry, E., Barrett, G. and Victor, C.R. (1999) Changes in household composition of the over sixties: a longitudinal analysis of the Health and Lifestyle Survey, *Health and Soical Care in the Community*, 7(2): 109–19.

Phillipson, C., Bernard, M., Phillips, J. and Ogg, J. (2001) *Family and Community Life of Older People*. London: Routledge.

Shah, S. and Cook, D.G. (2001) Inequalities in the treatment and control of hypertension: age, social isolation and lifestyle are more important than economic circumstances, *Journal of Hypertension*, 19: 1333–40.

Sheldon, J.H. (1948) *The Social Medicine of Old Age*. Oxford: Oxford University Press.

Townsend, P. (1957) *The Family Life of Old People*. London: Routledge & Kegan Paul.

Tunstall, J. (1966) *Old and Alone*. London: Routledge and Kegan Paul.

Victor, C.R., Scambler, S., Bond, J. and Bowling, A. (2001) Has loneliness amongst older people increased since 1945? Paper presented at British Society of Gerontology Annual Conference, Stirling University, September.

5

Using the Mass-Observation Archive

Dorothy Sheridan

Introduction

This chapter focuses on a particular historical resource, the Mass-Observation Archive (MOA) at the University of Sussex (see website address in Appendix). This archive offers not only rich survey and observational data on the life course and the experience of ageing during the mid- to late twentieth century but also continues to act as a centre for the collection of autobiographical accounts of everyday life in the present day. The original 'Mass-Observation' was an independent and pioneering research organization which operated between 1937 and the early 1950s. The papers resulting from its activities were brought to the university in 1970 after having been rescued from an office basement in London and they have been available as a public archive ever since.

   The relaunch in 1981, using the archive as the administrative base, was the first exploratory attempt to revive at least some of the original ideas of Mass-Observation. It was carried out by David Pocock, at that time Professor of Social Anthropology at Sussex, and Dorothy Sheridan, the collection's archivist. At the heart of this new Mass-Observation project was the recruitment of people from all over Britain to produce a collective account of everyday life in their own words which would complement the earlier documentation in the archive. This new phase of Mass-Observation, which has now been running almost continuously for twenty years, is rooted in the ideas and practices of the original Mass-Observation (Calder 1985; Summerfield 1985; Stanley 1990; Jeffery 1999; Sheridan *et al.* 2000).

Mass-Observation 1937–55

We are continually impressed by the discrepancy between what is supposed to happen and what does happen, between law and fact, the institution and the individual, what people say they do and what they actually do, what leaders think people want and what people do want.

(Madge and Harrisson 1938: 32)

The idea of conducting a detailed study of everyday life in Britain grew out of discussions between a group of young friends living in London in 1936. They chose the name 'Mass-Observation' to denote a popular form of social research, more democratic and participatory than other forms, one which would address issues of real interest to the general public and make its findings available to 'ordinary' people and which, most significantly, would involve the 'masses' as writers of their own history. They described it as 'anthropology at home'. Mass-Observation was therefore born out of a desire to experiment with anthropology: to observe and record the trivial, the inconsequential, the routine, the very intimate, and the domestic, to raise awareness about things otherwise taken for granted. They set out to subject the ordinary people of London, or Manchester or Glasgow, to the same anthropological scrutiny as that which had been applied to the peoples of far-off exotic islands by adventurer–anthropologists from Europe or North America.

The special interest of data from this early period for the study of ageing and later life is that it includes a large collection of autobiographical or life writings. These take the form of diaries on the one hand, and detailed personal replies to thematic open-ended questionnaires on the other. They maintained what they called an unpaid 'national panel' of writers all over the country who corresponded with the central organization, many of them well into the 1950s.

About 500 members of this national panel kept daily diaries which they sent to Mass-Observation in monthly instalments. Very few instructions were given about how to write these diaries and as a result they vary enormously in length and in degree of personal detail. Some of them have been edited for publication (see Broad and Fleming 1981; Sheridan 1985 1990) and plans to publish more diaries are underway. A large number of the panel agreed to respond to 'directives' or open-ended questionnaires which Mass-Observation sent to them every month. The questions usually elicited detailed thematic responses which are easier to analyse than the diaries. Lists of the themes covered between 1939 and 1955 can be obtained from the Mass-Observation website as can detailed catalogues of the papers resulting from the observations and surveys. Ageing as a distinct subject was not studied but considerable information about the experience of growing old can be mined from almost any of the replies from older people on themes as varied as personal appearance, political attitudes, income, attitudes to war work, food habits, leisure pursuits, health, education, friendship, family, housing and so on. There is a database of the contributors which includes their date of birth; see website address in Appendix.

The enthusiasm of these non-expert contributors is apparent throughout the archive even though they were unpaid and unidentified (they remained anonymous to protect their privacy). They shared the same agenda as the founders of Mass-Observation, and participation gave many of them a feeling that their everyday lives were valued and of interest.

It would be fruitful not only to examine material in the archive written by people who were already older in the 1930s and 1940s but also to explore the writing of the younger participants as a way of understanding the subjectivities of people who comprise the present-day older generation and whose early life experiences were forged during these years of rapid social change.

After 1981: the Mass-Observation Project

The decision to start a collection of contemporary life writings was made in 1981. Could the original Mass-Observation ideas of the 1930s be revived in the context of the 1980s? Would people still be willing to write about their lives? It was a tentative and experimental start. There were no special funds to support the relaunch, and no particular expectation that what was being undertaken would work. Without a budget for advertising, letters were sent to the editors of national and local newspapers appealing for volunteers to take part in a new Mass-Observation project. A variety of publications, both the 'quality' press and the tabloids, were deliberately chosen, but not all the newspapers published the letter. As a result, an unplanned and uneven distribution of publicity around the country successfully recruited the first new Mass-Observers. Since then, waves of usually unsolicited publicity in the press, on radio or on television have ensured that people still hear about the Mass-Observation activities and the archive continues to receive letters, email messages and phone calls from people offering to take part.

The highest numbers of writers on the mailing list at any one time was 1200 which had grown from about 300 in our first year of operation. Since 1981 almost 3000 people have participated at some time or other, some for several years, some sporadically, joining and leaving as it suits them. In terms of the composition, the project attracts about three times more women than men, and a higher proportion of people aged over 40. Geographically, the spread has been good, with writers coming from Scotland, Northern Ireland and Wales as well as England. The class background is not easily summarized; in terms of occupational categories, there is a preponderance of white-collar workers, but further examination of the family histories shows that a large number of the writers have quite modest origins, and may have been born into working-class homes. One distinctive feature is the high numbers of writers, especially among the women, whose education has been disrupted through no fault of their own (see Sheridan *et al.* 2000).

New volunteers are sent a small booklet describing the project and inviting them to send in an autobiography as long or as short as they wish, and a photograph. It is explained that they will hear from the archive two or three times a year. If some people prefer to keep continuous personal diaries and send instalments at intervals to the archive, these are accepted, but most of the contemporary writers (known as correspondents) respond to a prompt, or series of prompts, sent to them at intervals by the archive. These prompts continue to be called 'directives' and, as used in the original phase of Mass-Observation, take the form of detailed, discursive open-ended questionnaires. They are designed to be thought-provoking, encouraging, self-disclosing, that is what most sociologists might consider as leading. The idea is to stimulate thinking and writing, to make people feel interested and stimulated into expressing their views and describing their experiences. There is a variation in the 'voice' used for the directives even when the same author (usually Sheridan) is writing them. This may be because of the nature of the subject matter itself or because there may be more than one 'directive author' as in the case of a collaborative or commissioned directive. For an example of a directive, see Figure 5.1.

What motivates the correspondents to take part?

There are many common themes to be found in the reasons people give for taking part in Mass-Observation and, as in any relationship, the rewards and meanings may shift over time. There is considerable evidence to show that the longer a person stays with the project, the greater their sense of loyalty and commitment. They talk of enjoying the writing, feeling it is helping them to develop their writing and thinking skills. They use the directive questions to stimulate their ideas, and sometimes to initiate discussions with other people or to convey information to other people who read what they write. Some of the older people talk of the directives keeping them alert and up to date with current events. Many people speak of sorting out their ideas, of planning their lives in the future, even of finding out what they feel. Unsurprisingly, there is a therapeutic or confessional element to some of the accounts. Mass-Observers who do other writing use the directive replies as a springboard or resource for their other creative activities.

The link between the Mass-Observation project and an educational institution is significant. For those people who see universities as progressive and influential places the archive's home at the university is an incentive to join. For some Mass-Observers the University of Sussex still evokes memories of its radical past in the 1960s. Ensuring that their ideas and

Celebrating
20 years of
the new
Mass-
Observation
Project
1981–2001

Part 1: Courting and dating

This part of the directive is intended to find out about your experiences of courtship and dating. You do not have to answer all of the questions or answer them in the same order. Please add any additional thoughts on courtship which we have not covered. If you don't have any personal experiences to recount, perhaps you could describe your views and thoughts on courting today and in the past. Please bear in mind that we are interested in both heterosexual and homosexual experiences, and it would be helpful if you made it clear whether your loved one is/was male or female.

What does the word 'courtship' mean to you?

> *As usual, please remember to start your reply with a very brief mini-biography: your M-O number, (NOT name), sex, age, marital status, town or village where you live and your occupation or former occupation.*

♥ What other words would you use to describe this type of behaviour?
♥ What were/are your criteria for the 'perfect' partner?
♥ What is your understanding of the concept 'love'?

Personal experiences of courtship
♥ How old were you when you first stated dating? Please make sure you say where you live/were living as we are particularly interested in uncovering regional differences in courtship behaviour.
♥ Did anybody try to control whom you could date and where you could go?
♥ Please describe the things you did when courting. Think very widely and include everything from dancing and cinema-going to just sitting and talking.
♥ On a date, who would pay for activities? Yourself, your partner or did you share?
♥ If your courtship ended in marriage (or a committed living together type of relationship)
   - how far into the relationship did you decide to marry/live together?
   - how many months/years did you date before marriage/living together?

- ♥ If your courtship led to you living with your partner, but not marrying, how many months/years did you date before moving in together?
- ♥ If you resumed courtship behaviour at a later stage in your life, how old were you, and how did the experience differ from earlier courting experiences?
- ♥ Have you ever used a matchmaker or have you ever acted as a matchmaker? Stories please.
- ♥ Was you marriage arranged? Please tell us about this. And whether courtship played any role.
- ♥ Have you ever been on a blind date and if so was it successful?
- ♥ Have you ever made use of a dating agency or escort agency?

Sex and Courtship
- ♥ What forms of physical intimacy did you think were/are appropriate for each stage of courtship?
- ♥ Have you ever ended a relationship because of a difference of opinion about the role of sex in courtship?

Courtship Today
- ♥ How do you think the behaviour of courting couples has changed over the course of your life?
- ♥ Do you think that your own courting experiences have influenced your attitude towards the courting activities of other family members?
- ♥ Do you have any experience of how electronic communication has changed courting behaviour (use of e-mail, dating via the web, chatrooms)? Do you think it might have superseded writing love letters?

If you have time, please add any other reflections or stories about courting or dating from your own experience.

Figure 5.1 Example of an MO directive

experiences are making a contribution to enlightened research is appealing and rewarding, even if the link to politics and policy changes is indirect. Indeed, for one woman in her eighties, simply being able to boast to her bossy social worker that she 'did work for Sussex University' was in a small way 'empowering' for her.

The other consequence of being based in an institution, particularly when it is called an 'archive', is the promise that the writing will receive the same care and research interest that other important archived historical documents receive, and that it will ensure the survival of the writing for the future. When asked what they got out of writing for Mass-Observation, most of the correspondents cited the promise of posterity as one of the rewards. This is particularly significant for older people. This holds true even without the possibility of publication although the Mass-Observers are aware that extracts from their material may be reproduced in books and journal articles. One woman said in an interview:

When I die I want to leave things. I don't want to just pop my clogs and they'll say well there she goes, cheerio, good-bye. I want them to say, well she wrote a book, she did this writing for Mass-Observation, she knitted me a lovely bedspread, things like that you know. I won't be able to leave any cooking behind will I? But you know, I'd like to think there's going to be a lot of me left really.

(Mass-Observer No. F1373 1993)

But even for these people academia may be seen as remote and out of touch. Their task, then, as informants, is to ensure that the collective record to which they contribute *is* worldly and *does* contain the languages and meanings of everyday life, whether that is from the world of an office, a prison, an oil rig or a school. This same view of the project may explain why some people do *not* volunteer for Mass-Observation. The university setting acts as a deterrent, either because potential writers are alienated from mainstream education or because they see a university and all it entails at best as an irrelevance and at worst as a bastion of élitism and conservatism. Even those people who volunteer to write, and enjoy doing so, are conscious of the privilege of a university both in terms of what it represents about social class and in terms of its geographical situation in the relatively more affluent south of England. This raises further questions about the exploitation of people's intellectual property and the problems of power differentials between the Mass-Observers and those who use their writing for research (see Shaw 1998 and Sheridan *et al.* 2000: 237–79).

So for many people, the Mass-Observation project will never hold much attraction, unless it were possible to mount very specific and probably face-to-face recruitment drives which link closely with the appropriate community and grassroots organizations. We know that writers take up specific social roles and identities in different cultural contexts (Barton and Ivanic 1991; Street 1993). In households, in workplaces, in communities, different people do different kinds of writing. Women in this society are more likely to be family 'archivists', to maintain social and family networks through personal letters, to keep all kinds of journals and diaries, and many are skilled at precisely this kind of writing. This helps explain why Mass-Observation is more likely to appeal to them, rather than to men, because it builds on, and even legitimates and extends, their existing practices. Further evidence of the gendered nature of writing is becoming evident as more men turn to electronic mail as a form of communication. In the future we may see a rise in the number of young men joining in the project because their enjoyment of using email allows them to feel comfortable about taking part in what otherwise might feel like 'women's writing'. It is very clear from our research on literacy practices that unless taking part in Mass-Observation is congruent with people's understandings of specific forms of literacy, they are unlikely to see the relevance or value of the activity for them. For this reason, it would be impossible to impose participation in a Mass-Observation-style project on categories of people just because these categories are under-represented in the Mass-Observation panel – a factor which obviously has crucial implications for any attempts to make the Mass-Observation panel statistically representative of the whole population.

The nature of the MOA material

There are similarities between the Mass-Observation project and other life history approaches, but there are also significant differences. Most oral history, for example, tends to focus on life review from one point in time (see Bornat, Chapter 8 in this volume). In the Mass-Observation project, not only are the same people encouraged to stay involved, but they are invited to contribute continuously. This has advantages for both the writers and the researchers. For the writers there is always the chance of reworking, or re-presenting their lives, of making clarifications, of describing change and contradiction; they get a second, and a third and a fourth chance. They are free to take the story in different directions, to explore for themselves different subjects, or even to reject a subject and criticize the way it has been expressed in the directive. The correspondents send in all kinds of additional material: letters, stories, poetry, cartoons, articles they have written – material which was not primarily written for the archive but which they come to feel they would like to have on record. They are free to write in short fragments, or in long discourses on their lives and viewpoints. There is no obligation to write large amounts, or to produce definitive statements. There is always another opportunity to write again.

The researcher is likely to be able to gain access to a greater degree of candour from the correspondents than that likely to emerge in an interview. The trust and commitment mentioned earlier facilitates openness. Things which could not be revealed at first (a notable example is confiding sexual preference, but also admissions of political affiliations) are possible to reveal in time and with the protection of anonymity. The absence of face-to-face contact, for some people, permits greater use of the imagination by the narrator, and enables people who are shy, or who do not wish to be identified, to be more open. For researchers interested in the subjective meanings which a person may make in his or her life, then this kind of access is highly valuable, even while it still must be understood as a representation, a particular version, told for a specific (imagined) audience and under specific historical conditions. They tell us *what they want to have documented*, not what we think should be documented. They see themselves not as subjects of research but as *partners* in research, contributing to a kind of collective documentation of life in Britain. As a result researchers enter into reciprocal obligations to respect the Mass-Observers but, at the same time, they benefit from what becomes a special and unusual relationship. It represents a variation of the kind of involvement of people in research, discussed by Peace (Chapter 14 in this volume).

Research use and interpretation

There are now some 2500 archival storage boxes of papers in the archive. About 2000 of these cover the period from 1937 to the 1950s, and a further 500 boxes cover the years 1981 to the present, arranged chrono-logically and by themes. They cover a wide range of national and international topical issues, including the Gulf War and 11 September 2001, as well as more personal issues such as home and family, health, education, music, dancing, hobbies, work, travel, sleep, holidays, children, death, birth, pleasure, marriage and love. For the researchers, the contemporary collection offers unparalleled access to the process of change and transformation in the life course at the micro level, and the opportunity to examine one life from many different angles, and over a period of time, in relation to the grander (macro) sweeps of social and economic change. Researchers using the archive are also encouraged to employ qualitative methods of analysis, for example, narrative or discourse analysis, a case study approach, close reading, grounded theory and analytic deduction. The increasing popularity of what has been termed the 'biographical turn' (Chamberlayne *et al.* 2000) in social research is providing the kind of literature in research methodologies which can be fruitfully used to interpret the Mass-Observation material.

The study of ageing and later life

This chapter has concentrated so far on the general features of the Mass-Observation enterprise. There are, however, some specific attributes which suggest that there is a special value in the material for scholars of the life course and ageing.

The greater numbers of older people on the panel

The project is especially successful at attracting and retaining people over 50 years of age. Of the 367 people on our mailing list at the moment, 236 or 64 per cent are over 50, 48 per cent are over 60, 33 per cent over 70 and 9 per cent are over 80. So what for many researchers is one of the weaknesses of the present-day panel, that is the preponderance of older people, becomes the strength of the research data in this field. The age profile of the earlier archive is younger, and many contributors have aged with the project.

The longitudinal nature of participation

Many of the people have been writing for several years. For example, four of the over-80s have taken part for the whole of the twenty years the project has been operating, and 14 of them have written continuously for more than 15 years, thus recording in considerable detail their thoughts and experiences as they grow older. Of people who continued to write until their deaths (we know for sure about 68 people because their relatives write to tell us) most were over 70 and several had been born in the nineteenth century. Their participation in the project was almost invariably for more than five years, and often over fifteen. Occasionally an older person resigns because it has become too hard for him or her physically to write, in which case we suggest speaking into a tape recorder, if one can be obtained. From time to time, people will say that they have become too old and their world too narrow to feel able to continue. In these cases I try to persuade them not to leave us and usually they are pleased to be persuaded. The project itself is a record of the ageing process over 20 years, whether someone goes from 32 to 52, or from 62 to 82, and if ageing is taken to mean the process of growing older at any point in one's life, then we have access here to a huge amount of information about the life span.

Description and redescriptions: layered life stories

The nature of the writing, at intervals throughout the years, makes the resulting document rather different from a life review or traditional autobiography. In a discussion about autobiography and life course, Luk Van Langenhove and Rom Harré argue against the monolithic idea of 'one life' told through the traditional vehicle of a literary model of autobiography. For research purposes, they see this autobiographical template as reified and commend what they call 'biographical talk', or orality, as being preferred. This is to enable people to create *redescriptions* of their lives. 'Life span research cannot thus simply take for granted the so widely spread idea in our western culture that we all have one biography' (Van Langenhove and Harré 1993: 97). I would argue that this capacity to describe and *redescribe* is not a discursive practice limited to oral communication, but is apparent within the writings of the Mass-Observers, who over many years may reinvent themselves and their biographies, telling the same stories from different angles (depending on the theme of the directive) or different stories at different stages of their life. This enables us to have access to the contradictions of everyday life, and to the changes in people's perceptions of themselves and the world they inhabit. Rather than base our research on a one-off cross section, a moment frozen in time or a retrospective account which offers a rather different perspective on a life, we can wend our way through the complications of living, through what are layered life stories, told at different times, with different emphases, and mixing what happened today with what happened 30, 40, 50 years ago.

The subject matter of the writing

It is particularly invidious to suggest themes of relevance to the study of ageing because it is easy to stereotype the preoccupations of older people, to stress issues such as physical deterioration, or to choose topics assumed to be the province of people after retirement. A narrow focus would suggest directives with the following titles:

Growing older
The pace of life
Staying well in everyday life
Death and bereavement
Work
The NHS (50 years old)
Gardening
A wider trawl might include:
Pleasure
Music and dancing
Close relationships
Holidays
Travel
New technology
Food
Body images
Plans for the future
Gender
Extramarital affairs
Courting and dating (see Figure 5.1 . . .)

as well as themes on current events: political events and developments, general elections, wars, famine, disasters and issues such as racism, sexism, environmental questions, belief systems and so on.

The participatory nature of the project

As discussed earlier, the imbalance of power between researcher and re-searched cannot be abolished but it is to some extent mitigated by the extent to which the writers are able to use the project for their own ends and rewards and the ways in which they can use the writing as a form of empowerment. This has a special resonance for research into a traditionally invisible and powerless social group: older people. The very fact that their stories are used for research, and the processes of making sense of what is told, or claiming significance from it, by another person, underlines the value of these stories and thereby validates the process of recording and writing. The interpretation and analysis become an integral part of the original endeavour. The writers write to make a contribution to human understanding (not that they actually say it quite like that!). Theory making is not restricted to the academics involved. The story telling can itself be theorized by the writers in the process of writing. The writers work towards becoming *participants in* research rather than *subjects of* research.

The Archive constitutes an enormous data collection about how people grow older and about older people's lives written over the last twenty years of the twentieth century, some of it about the here and now, much of it recollecting the past, mixing together as the themes suggest or according to temperament and experience. What unites this collection is that it is from the point of view of the writers themselves. The modes of communication which people select from a culturally determined repertoire in order to take part in Mass-Observation suggest that there is some evidence of an M-O 'genre' emerging which draws on the family letter, the school essay, the newspaper report, the personal diary, the testimony and the confessional.

Future possibilities: work in progress

There are three areas of interconnected development which are desirable for the future: the diversification and extension of the panel membership; the continued creation of new directives in collaboration with interested (and preferably funded) scholars; and the further automation of the database to make analysis and retrieval of the material more efficient.

For the moment, the project has a momentum of its own but at some point soon, attention must be given to further recruitment. By the year 2002 the numbers in the panel had reduced to 350 although many of those who leave are replaced by new recruits, often contacting us (and continuing to contribute) by electronic mail via our appeal on the archive's website. In order to improve age range of the panel, a restriction on the numbers of new writers over the age of 50 has been imposed. People over 50 are not turned away; rather than join the main panel, they are invited to start a daily diary and to send it in on an annual basis. While recognizing that the panel can never be fully representative, there is scope for extending the diversity of the writers and this could be an area of fruitful development. It has become clear that the methods of recruitment used in the past (publicity in the national media) have not been as effective as they could have been in attracting certain categories of people, young men especially, people from Asian and African-Caribbean communities and working-class writers. Different ways of reaching people need to be developed but this would have to be preceded by strenuous fundraising efforts as there is currently no budget to fund such activities.

One source of financial support has in the past been collaboration with academic colleagues who have obtained funding for their research. Researchers who wish to define their own questions or for whom there is no relevant material already in the archive have approached Sheridan with ideas for collaboration, and a number of the directives have been conceived jointly with researchers, among others on topics such as gardening practices, body images and shopping.

The constant demand by students and academic researchers for access to the collection which has already been accumulated increases pressure on our systems of analysis and retrieval. Further automation of the database is overdue; biographical information (including date of birth) is currently recorded on a database (MS ACCESS) and this allows for address label printing for the mailing of directives to the writers and facilitates administrative 'housekeeping'. Basic biographical analysis is therefore possible. However, the information about what the individual Mass-Observer writes and which directive he or she replies to is still recorded only on a manual card index. This information, now accumulated over twenty years, urgently needs to be converted into electronic form. The possibilities of digitizing the whole collection remain a further possibility but this would be enormously expensive and until electronic methods are developed to handle a variety of different handwritten texts, the benefits of an electronic resource remain questionable in relation to the costs.

Meanwhile, the boxes of papers continue to be consulted every day at the archive. They provide a resource for scholars working in anthropology, social psychology, sociology, history, art history, media studies and feminist studies. They are used as a resource in the teaching and learning of research epistemologies and methodologies at both undergraduate and postgraduate levels, for example in the Masters course at Sussex on life history research; they are explored as narrative texts by linguists and literature specialists and by novelists, poets and playwrights hungry for creative ideas about everyday life and language. They are read as inspiration for their own projects by schoolchildren and teachers, by writers' groups and community groups, and they remain, as far as I am aware, the only collection of its kind in Britain, and one of the few in the world to give pride of place to the *written* testimonies of 'ordinary' people.

References

Barton, D. and Ivanic, R. (eds) (1991) *Writing in the Community*. Newbury Park: Sage Publications.

Calder, A. (1985) Mass-Observation 1937–49, in M. Bulmer (ed.) *Essays on the History of British Sociological Research*, Cambridge: Cambridge University Press.

Chamberlayne, P., Bornat, J. and Wengraf, T. (eds) (2000) *The Turn to Biographical Methods in Social Science*. London: Routledge.

Jeffery, T. (1999) *Mass-Observation: A Short History*, Mass-Observation Archive occasional paper no. 10. Brighton: University of Sussex.

Madge, C. and Harrisson, T. (1938) *First Year's Work by Mass-Observation*. London: Lindsay Drummond.

Shaw, J. (1998) *Intellectual Property, Representative Experience and Mass-Observation*, Mass-Observation Archive occasional paper no. 9. Brighton: University of Sussex.

Sheridan, D., Street, B.V. and Bloome, D. (2000) *Writing Ourselves: Mass-Observation and Literacy Practices*. Cresskill, NJ: Hampton Press.

Stanley, L. (1990) *The Archeology of a 1930s Mass-Observation Project*, occasional paper no. 27. Manchester: Department of Sociology, University of Manchester.

Street, B. (ed.) (1993) *Cross-cultural Approaches to Literacy*. Cambridge: Cambridge University Press.

Summerfield, P. (1985) Mass-Observation: Social Research or Social Movement?, *Journal of Contemporary History*, 20: 439–52.

Van Langenhove, L. and Harré, R. (1993) Positioning and autobiography: telling your life, in N. Coupland and J. Nussbaum (eds) *Discourse and Life Span Identity*. Thousand Oaks, CA: Sage Publications.

Using 'cultural products' in researching images of ageing

Mike Hepworth

Definitions

In this chapter I shall define cultural products as the images available to us to make sense of the experiences of ageing.

The term 'cultural products' clearly indicates that images of ageing are the products of human imaginative activities which reflect the beliefs and values of the particular historical periods during which they were made. This can be illustrated by two examples of visual images selected from classical antiquity: the image of Old Silenus offering a bowl of wine to a young satyr in a wall painting on the Hall of Mysteries at Pompeii and the marble statue from Ancient Greece of the Old Fisherman. The former is evidence of the level of technical accomplishment of the artists of the time and a representation of a set of religious beliefs and practices which are far removed from present-day life. Old Silenus, crowned in vine leaves, is not simply the only older figure among a group of youthful men and women but his appearance of age reflects the particular symbolic role he has to play in the pre-Christian ritual recorded in the mural (Nappo 1998). We can examine this image, therefore, with a number of questions in mind: the level of technical competence; the style of representation of Old Silenus; his relationship to the younger figures; and the specific symbolic significance of this image of old age in the religious beliefs that these murals celebrate. We can then relate our knowledge to the present-day cultural context and contemporary ways of creating, perceiving, and interpreting images of later life.

A similar range of factors have to be taken into account when attempting to understand the meaning of the statue of Old Fisherman (Stewart 1997). In addition to our appreciation of the technical skill evident in the meticulous carving of the wrinkles and folds of his almost naked body, and the lines of the ageing bearded face, we can try to discover the significance of this work for the people for whom it was actually made. On one level the Old Fisherman needs no explanation: it is immediately recognizable to us today as the body of an older man. But if we wish to put him into historical context, we need to look for evidence concerning the viewpoint of the ancient Greeks. We can discover that Greek scholars argue that the contemporary meaning can be traced to the high value placed on images of the athletic body of the youthful male which were prominent symbols of military and political power (Stewart 1997). This statue of the Old Fisherman derives its meaning to the Greeks from their direct contrast with sculptures of the vigorous and tautly muscled male body with which we, as present-day viewers, are much more familiar.

These two examples suggest five questions we can ask when researching any kind of cultural product:

1 the level of technical skill displayed (sculpture, painting, engraving, writing);
2 the kind of images produced (sculpture, subject painting, portrait, play, film, TV drama, biography);
3 the aims of those who made the images (religious, political, financial, personal, self-expressive);
4 the location of the image (domestic wall painting, church, gallery, museum, library, newspaper);
5 the historical beliefs of the time when the images were produced and evidence of subsequent changes in perceptions of images and ageing.

Inevitably our ability to find answers to these questions will depend on the cultural products we select; the historical period; access to archival and other resources, and funding, and we cannot expect to find adequate evidence in all cases. For example, evidence of the intentions of an artist or author when dealing with later life is not always available and speculation is unavoidable. But they should always be kept in mind to qualify any observations and conclusions we may reach. In the rest of this chapter I shall concentrate on one source of evidence relatively accessible to anyone who wishes to research images of ageing: fiction, namely novels and short stories.

Before looking more closely at researching the cultural production of ageing in the novel a further point should be made about the symbolic nature of cultural products. As a biological species human beings are unique in their dependency on images to give meaning to life; such is our dependency on cultural products that Margaret Gullette, a leading American student of fictional images of ageing, has argued that 'whatever happens in the body, human beings are aged by culture first of all' (1997: 3). In her view fiction is an important resource for making sense of the everyday experiences of growing older (Humphrey 1993; Freeman 1997).

Recognition of the symbolic nature of cultural products inevitably brings the problem of *interpretation*. If, as I suggested in my reference to the two images of ageing from classical antiquity, the *meanings* of images are subject to historical change, our research must take into account possible variations in the ways they are perceived by different audiences. A good example is the increasing sensitivity to gender differences in ageing in gerontology. The symbolic construction of meaning expressed in visual and textual forms is never value-free and ageing in particular has always been interpreted as a moral process (Hepworth 1995). A good example is the value currently invested in Britain in the *image* of the Queen Mother who, like Queen Victoria before her, has come to symbolize an entire generation and a particularly 'British' way of life: the image of the Queen Mother is a national symbol of positive ageing (Hepworth 1995; on Queen Victoria see Homans and Munich 1997).

Cultural research does require a careful assessment of value judgements, but when the findings are carefully related to evidence from other gerontological research it helps to uncover the processes through which ageing is invested with personal and social significance, thereby furthering our understanding of the way ageing is constructed out of an interplay between the psychological, the sociological and the cultural.

Furthermore, cultural research helps us to understand the problematic relationship between fact and fiction in social life. Gerontology, like any form of knowledge, is itself a symbolic construct made possible by our use of language or discourse, a point made by Stephen Katz in his observation that gerontological knowledge is built out of an interplay between science and non-science: science 'borrows' from the wider culture metaphors and images of ageing including fiction (1996: 91). For Constance Rooke, who has examined images of ageing in novels such as Margaret Laurence's *The Stone Angel* ([1964] 1987), fiction is 'responsive to and constitutive of social realities' (1992: 242). In her analysis of the emergence of a more positive imagery of older people in the novel she argues that themes in fiction 'naturally overlap with themes that have interested gerontologists' (1992: 254). Among these she includes family conflict, disengagement, the life review, body image, sexuality, loss and death (1992: 254). And in her study of fictional representations of midlife, *Safe At Last in the Middle Years*, Margaret Gullette (1988) shows how gerontological thinking about ageing is shaped by cultural resources; there is no clear-cut boundary separating the social scientist's concern with the 'facts' of ageing from the cultural repertoire which we draw on to give those facts meaning. The key question we are asking in cultural analysis is 'what does it mean to grow old?' (Cole and Gadow 1986).

These questions make cultural research particularly challenging. If the meanings of images vary and are open to a variety of interpretations then research into images offers us an opportunity to search for evidence of the diversity, complexity and ambiguity that many gerontologists regard as characteristic of the ageing process (Bond, *et al.* 1993). Such evidence is essentially complementary to data resulting from the alternative forms of enquiry described in the other chapters of this book.

Range of practice in this field

Having discussed important general questions concerning research into cultural products I now turn to specific questions concerning research into images of ageing in fiction, a field of enquiry often described in the academic literature as 'literary gerontology' (Wyatt-Brown 1992a).

Anne Wyatt-Brown, a leading American researcher in the field, provides a concise review of the history of literary gerontology since the mid 1970s which saw the first stirrings of the discipline in America (1992a). One of the most important points she raises concerns the interdisciplinary nature of the research. The first task is to *read widely*: the analysis of ageing fiction must be done with reference to gerontological theory and practice.

I will illustrate this with an example from my own research. A few years ago I did a study of older people in Richmal Crompton's short stories about *William*, the incorrigible schoolboy whose adventures have entertained readers of all ages since she published her first story in 1919 (Hepworth 1996). I read (or reread) her stories and biography, discussed the issue with members of the William Society and then, having accumulated examples of older characters, compared her treatment with the theory of the infantilization of older people as developed in Hockey and James's study of negative attitudes towards older people (1993). As a result of this comparative reading of wide sources I was able to gather cultural evidence that infantilization – treating older people as if they are children – is not always a negative process and may under certain circumstances be interpreted as positive ageing. There are certain older characters in the *William* stories who are treated with approval because they are able to identify with children and behave in a 'childish' manner.

Data for the literary gerontologist are, of course, written texts and the analysis is qualitative because it requires an in-depth reading of stories together with biographical and critical publications if they are available. It is qualitative because it focuses on the fine detail of the subjective and interpersonal processes of ageing. In the case of Richmal Crompton, the *William* books are for the most part short stories so it is important to examine her brief character studies of older people in the context of the events and social encounters within which they are portrayed. But there are also large numbers of novels, for example Isler's *The Prince of West End Avenue* ([1994] 1996), where the central character is an older person and the narrative relates his/her subjective perception of life. As with other forms of research the nature of the findings is inevitably shaped by the nature of the data available, namely the kind of stories we are investigating in our research.

For my research into images of ageing in popular fiction (Hepworth 2000) I read a large number of novels published in Britain and America during the period 1930 to the present day. One of my aims was to try to discover the range of differences in the treatment of ageing by novelists and I came up with the following five variations. These must be regarded as provisional because much more work needs to be done.

1 *The interest of the writer is in one central character, often the narrator, who is ageing* (examples are diverse and include murder mysteries such as Anthony Gilbert's *The Spinster's Secret* ([1946] 1987) , Vita Sackville-West's pioneering feminist critique of marriage, *All Passion Spent* ([1931] 1989), and Henry Sutton's study of older people living in retirement at the seaside, *Gorleston* (1995)).
2 *A small group of older people living together* (includes hotels – Elizabeth Taylor's *Mrs Palfrey at The Claremont* ([1971] 1996) and residential care – Kathleen Conlon's *Face Values* ([1985] 1986), Alan Isler's *The Prince of West End Avenue* ([1994] 1996)).
3 *Processes of family interaction* (includes studies of middle-class family life where a concern is inheritance, like Nina Bawden's *Family Money* (1997) – also dramatized for television – and Pat Barker's sensitive story of working-class life and the problems of ageing for poorer women, *The Century's Daughter* (1986)).
4 *Age-related interaction outside the family situation* (includes Barbara Ewing's *The Actresses* (1997) dealing largely with the lives of actresses who are growing older, and Stanley Middleton's *Beginning to End* (1991)).
5 *The appearances of older people tend to be incidental or situational* – ageing is not the main interest of the story as such but descriptions of older people and the ageing process may play a significant part of the story when they are used for dramatic effect or to give the impression of social realism, for example a village community or the human diversity of an urban scene (the range is enormous and includes Colin Dexter's *The Wench is Dead* ([1989] 1990), James Herriot's *If Only They Could Talk* (1970) and Laurie Lee's *Cider With Rosie* (1962)).

For the purposes of my research, evidence from stories in all five variations in the treatment of ageing was valuable because I was able to use these different materials to exemplify and develop my reading of the symbolic interactionist analysis in social gerontology. I was therefore able to compare these fictional examples with findings from gerontological research in Britain and America and to use symbolic interactionism as my conceptual framework for the interpretation of a wide diversity of stories of ageing.

Having selected the kind of fiction to be researched (for example crime fiction, romantic fiction, poetry, the work of a particular author such as Dickens, the Brontës, or in work I am currently doing on the fiction of Stanley Middleton (Hepworth, forthcoming)), it is necessary, as I have noted previously, to determine its gerontological relevance; in other words, to answer the question: why am I doing this research? We can find help with this by referring to the aims of literary gerontologists. These may be summarized as follows.

Unmasking or exposing ageism and the crude one-dimensional stereotyping of older people

This includes description of the power struggles in later life in, for example, residential care where there is a struggle on the part of the older central character for the preservation of the self. Examples are May Sarton's famous novel of one woman's negative experiences of residential care, *As We Are Now* ([1973] 1992), which assumes an added richness when read alongside her autobiographical writings on her own ageing in, for example, her journal, *At Eighty-Two* (1996), and Paul Bailey's *At The Jerusalem* (1987): a novel showing how the individual identity of the main character, again a woman, is put in jeopardy when she has to enter The Jerusalem for residential care.

Other examples include Kehl's (1988) thematic analysis of 25 poems and nine works of fiction by 35 modern authors (American, British, Australian, French) which argues that belletristic literature (defined as literature 'dealing with what it means to be human' (1988: 1)) exposes crude stereotypes and offers a fuller reading of individual character. This literature avoids 'conventional, oversimplified, formulaic, superficial images or conceptions that lack critical judgement and individualising characteristics ... [which] are a common mechanism for avoiding authentic responses to such human experiences as ageing, and particularly the ageing of women' (1988: 2). Kehl's selection includes Barbara Pym's *Quartet in Autumn* ([1977] 1994) (Britain); May Sarton's *As We Are Now* ([1973] 1992) (America); Elizabeth Taylor's *Mrs Palfrey at The Claremont* ([1971] 1996) (Britain); Patrick White's *The Eye of the Storm* (1975) (Australia).

But, as Richard Freedman (1978) has warned, we have to be careful about the idea that fiction necessarily adopts a critical approach to popular stereotypes. In a famous article he criticizes the assumption that great literature necessarily displays older people in a positive or sympathetic light. In examples chosen from a wide variety of texts including Shakespeare, Jane Austen and Arnold Bennett he shows a significant thread of 'literary gerontophobia' (1978: 51) running through influential plays and novels.

Fostering a humanistic approach to ageing and later life: the idea that literature is concerned with individual self-development and the rich variations in the individual experience of ageing

Unlike Freedman, the majority of researchers favour a humanistic perspective on ageing which looks for ways of giving positive value to the experience of growing older. There are a number of collections of selections from literary works with this aim including Cole and Winkler's *Oxford Book of Ageing* (1994).

In terms of sustained analysis of specific authors, Margaret Gullette (1988) has published a detailed study of Saul Bellow, Margaret Drabble, Anne Tyler, and John Updike.

Exploring creativity in mid- and later life: fiction is seen as a resource for both writers and readers

Anne Wyatt-Brown's studies of creative writing in later life include her book-length study of Barbara Pym (1992b) and papers on E.M. Forster and Virginia Woolf (1989a), and Anita Brookner (1989b).

She shows that a significant number of novels written by middle-aged authors are autobiographical: 'Literary manuscripts suggest that middle-age can provide an important creative turning point' (1989b: 176). It is possible to see how a reading of a number of novels by the same author can show how his or her attitude to ageing is changing and developing. After a decline in popularity the English novelist Barbara Pym returned to public favour with *Quartet in Autumn* ([1977]1994), a novel about four retired people published when she was 64, forged 'out of illness and the threat of approaching death' (Wyatt-Brown 1992b: 124). Pym had discovered she was suffering from cancer and *Quartet* can be read with the insights of gerontology as a 'test (of) three current theories about retirement: abandonment, liberation and what sociologists call "diachronic solidarity"' (1992b: 124).

Gullette observes in *Safe At Last* that writing 'life course fiction' might 'assist personal transformation' in midlife (1988: xxvi) and reading such fiction can facilitate self-analysis which can be conducive to positive ageing. In *Declining to Decline* she says that her seminars encourage women students to read fictions about women in midlife in order to discover what kind of information each person *casually* absorbed from 'normal readings' (1988: 236).

The promotion of new agendas for positive ageing: new ways of coping with change expressed in efforts to create new vocabularies and images of later life

Key examples are Gullette's pathbreaking work on midlife (1988) and her critical engagement with the 'decline narrative' of later life in her *Declining to Decline* (1997).

In their edited collection of 250 works Cole and Winkler argue that later life in present-day society is 'a season in search of its purposes'(1994: 3). Social change has resulted in a situation where ideas about ageing have changed dramatically and we are now living at a time when people 'have become deeply uncertain about what it means to grow old' (1994: 3).

Descriptions of variations in the experience of ageing according to family membership, gender, social status, and ethnicity

Examples include novels which focus on women's experiences of ageing, some of which include aspects of social class such as Pat Barker's *The Century's Daughter* (1986) and Jane Smiley's *At Paradise Gate* ([1981]1995); an example of a novel which is grounded in aspects of cultural identity is Alan Isler's *The Prince of West End Avenue* ([1994] 1996). In an exemplary doctoral thesis on fiction and ageing Hannah Zeilig (1999) has sensitively explored ageing and family interaction in a number of novels published in England during the interwar period including Vita Sackville-West's *All Passion Spent* ([1931] 1989), Hugh Walpole's *The Old Ladies* (1927) and John Galsworthy's The Forsyte Saga (1942).

When making decisions about the selection of material, the gerontological issues of concern, and questions of interpretation outlined above, it is most important to remember that the primary concern of this kind of research is not literary (although literary criticism may be an invaluable resource) or aesthetic. Questions of literary value (whether a novel, for example, is considered an example of 'high' or 'popular' culture) are of less interest than the information that may be gathered about attitudes to ageing, the range of variations in the experience of ageing, the place of a particular work within the history of ideas, and evidence of cultural intersections of fiction with other forms of writing about ageing.

Case studies

To illustrate some of the issues raised above I now give brief gerontological interpretations of the content of **two** novels selected from the popular genre of crime fiction. These stories cannot be described technically as novels about ageing as such; they are first and foremost murder mysteries, written as entertainments, but ageing plays a significant part in the narrative and we can interpret these passages in terms of the aims of literary gerontology and questions to guide our research outlined above.

Case study 1: *Anthony Gilbert,* The Spinster's Secret*

'Anthony Gilbert' was the pen-name of Lucy Beatrice Malleson. Her crime story, first published in [1946] 1987, centres around the last months in the life of Janet Martin, the spinster of the title (Hepworth 1993). Having devoted the best years of her life to looking after her invalid mother (a period touch indicated in the use of the word 'spinster' in the title), she is now aged 74 and, although suffering from some of the physical frailties associated with later life, is mentally sound. She has weak eyes, receives few letters, and is without relatives except for a niece whom she sees occasionally and an affluent married nephew who lives in the north and has 'no time for the unsuccessful' ([1946] 1987: 2). She passes the day observing the social scene from the window of her bed-sitting room in Blakely House which offers privately rented sheltered accommodation. Blakely House is presided over by the formidable Miss Fraser who believes in adopting a brisk manner with old ladies who otherwise would lapse into 'self-pity, and everyone knew that was fatal' ([1946] 1987: 3). The threat of expulsion is, therefore, an ever-present sanction.

Although this novel was written shortly after the Second World War and therefore has a distinctly 'period' feel about it (on one level it can be read as a glimpse into one facet of social history), we can also see that Gilbert's description of Miss Martin's situation and the ageism with which she is surrounded is congruent with more contemporary gerontological analyses.

Miss Martin's other pleasure in life is derived from wandering through the streets and observing the activities of those around her. In her interest in observation she shares one of the chief characteristics of Agatha Christie's Miss Marple whose gendered position in detective fiction has been closely scrutinized by Craig and Cadogan (1981), and Shaw and Vanacker (1991). The first part of the story, seen through her own eyes, is therefore about Miss Martin's discovery of her 'secret' (which is that a murder has been committed) and her attempts to persuade others that this is the case. The reader is invited to share her knowledge of a truth to which others are blind largely because their vision is obscured by an ageist stereotype of elderly spinsters as feeble-minded. All her efforts to communicate her suspicions are received unsympathetically and simply confirm the suspicions of those around her, including professional carers, that she is becoming

---

* This discussion first appeared in Hepworth, M. (2000) *Stories of Ageing.* Buckingham: Open University Press.

senile. Already regarded as 'odd' by her middle-aged niece, she is removed from Blakely House and admitted to Beverley, 'advertised as a Rest-Home for ladies requiring light attention and care' ([1946] 1987: 25).

At Beverley she is forced into close and unwelcome contact with 'desiccated' older women. At tea 'she met her room-mate, a distinctly eccentric old lady, who enlivened the nights by suddenly starting up and crying that they must get ready, for the day of the Lord was at hand, and asking Miss Martin if she too could not see signs and portents in the sky' ([1946] 1987: 28). As readers are fully aware, Miss Martin's problem is that those who 'care' for her are prevented by their stereotyped theories of ageing into old age from recognizing the truth of her claims and distinguishing her from other older people whose perceptions are more impaired. The author's use of a conventional narrative device enables readers to share her dilemma and frustration; we identify with Miss Martin in the same way that qualitative researchers in gerontology set out to identify with the subjective perspective of their older interviewees.

As the story unfolds Miss Martin makes increasingly urgent efforts to confirm her suspicions and to find evidence to support the reality of her claims. She tries unobtrusively to observe what she believes to be the scene of the murder (a location that appears to others to be a commonplace and innocent private house), and is in turn observed by the doctor's wife who lives in the house opposite. This observer of the observed simply concludes that Miss Martin is an 'old thing' who is completely unaware of 'the daft appearance she presented, with bits of twigs in her hair and her hat askew' as 'she went pattering down the road at a great rate' ([1946] 1987: 73).

As when reading qualitative gerontological research, the reader of this novel is privileged because s/he has access to two perspectives on reality. The story opens with the view from Miss Martin and the promise (since this story is a murder mystery) of her vindication. Because she is an exceptional older woman (she is the only other older character in the book who is not 'desiccated' or senile), she is at once a testimony to the power of the stigma of ageing (the view from the outside) and counter-evidence of the distorted perception of the 'reality' of ageing that the stigma can produce. Her persistent attempts to discover evidence (data) to substantiate her hypothesis are perceived by the younger characters as cumulative evidence of her age-induced eccentricity. The doctor who professionally examines Miss Martin after his wife has seen her watching the house opposite shares this popular theory of the effects of ageing. In his experience many older people become 'queer' and the 'best place for senile cases was the institution, unless there was some convenient relative'. He is ready and willing to 'sign her up' and anticipates 'no difficulty in getting his opinion confirmed by another local doctor' ([1946] 1987: 116–17).

To summarize: as a novel published in the postwar 1940s this can be read as a historical document recording in descriptive detail, forms of speech and characterization the norms and expectations of the period. As such it offers interesting information about contemporary society. Equally, and rather like the example of the Greek statue of the Old Fisherman, we can see significant similarities with present-day attitudes towards older people and assumptions about the mental competencies of individuals as they grow older. We can also see how mistaken those assumptions can be and the problems they create for the maintenance of individual dignity and self-esteem. In terms of these two criteria Gilbert's novel helps us to relate the past to the present by shedding light on the social processes through which the 'burden' of ageing is socially constructed. It is therefore more than a murder mystery; it enlarges our humanistic understanding of ageing.

Case study 2: Peter Robinson, In a Dry Season

This novel is a good example of the value for the novelist of a chronological perspective in constructing a mystery and adding dramatic value to a story: in this case the discovery of a mysterious death sixty years ago. This narrative device permits an interplay between the past and present and the use of older people as suspects and possible witnesses. By using these two ploys the author can explore assumptions about ageing and its effects on memory and the effects of time passing on shaping identity.

As the title suggests, the mystery emerges when a drought drains a reservoir and exposes the remains of the Yorkshire village Hobb's End, flooded after the Second World War. An unknown skeleton is discovered by a young boy out playing in a derelict property. A key character is Vivian Elmsley, now a famous crime writer who was brought up in the village and is portrayed in later life as a mentally vigorous and creative individual.

Vivian Elmsley is significant because she is not a stereotypical older woman and her home is described as deliberately furnished in a contemporary minimalist style to avoid any identification with old age:

> Most people would have been surprised at the modern chrome-and-glass décor in the home of a person as old as Vivian, but she far preferred it to all the dreadfully twee antiques, knick-knacks and restored woodwork that cluttered up most old people's houses – at least the ones she had seen.
>
> ([1999] 2000: 28)

Her appearance, too, is described as unlike the typical older woman, though in one passage she looks at her hands after a book signing and notes they were 'the first to go' although 'the rest of her was remarkably well preserved. For a start, she had remained tall and lean. She hadn't shrunk or run to fat like so many elderly women, or generated that thick, matronly carapace' ([1999] 2000: 18). But she is not well preserved through the use of cosmetic surgery or other interventions. Her resistance to ageing is essentially intellectual: reading and creative writing. Robinson's description of her face signals this attitude to ageing:

> Steel-grey hair pulled back tightly and fastened at the back created a widow's peak over her strong, thin face; her deep blue eyes, networked with crow's-feet, were almost oriental in their slant, her nose was slightly hooked and her lips thin. Not a face that smiles often, people thought. And they were right, even though it had not always been so.
>
> ([1999] 2000: 19)

A description suggesting a strong character and also hinting at a past history or younger self that has been lost or masked by subsequent events. Ageing here helps to give this character a hint of mystery: there is, it is implied, more to her than meets the eye.

In a Dry Season is a superb example of the novelist's use of a number of images of ageing in the service of a murder mystery. In the process he enriches images of ageing and widens the range of different modes of ageing. Some of these images are incidental to creating a 'realistic' social landscape but others deliberately exploit conventional stereotypes for creative effect while at the same time opening up the ageing process to wider possibilities. As with *The Spinster's Secret* the gerontologist can read this novel on a number of levels: because of the chronological perspective, ranging from Yorkshire village life in the Second World War through to the contemporary social landscape, we obtain corroborative evidence of the situated nature of the ageing process, its variability and the patterning of intergenerational relationships.

Further research

While the guidelines for research into 'literary gerontology' are arguably more established than is the case, for example, with visual images such as paintings, a great deal of work still remains to be done. One reason for this window of opportunity can be found in the belief we tend to hold in the existence of wide variations in the subjective experience of ageing and the difficulty of obtaining data on the personal meanings of ageing through the utilization of conventional research techniques such as questionnaires. Much, it is therefore argued, is missing from the equation but this needs to be shown to be the case and substantiated as more than a pious hope. In other words, gerontology requires much more research into what is at the moment largely speculative territory. Because meaning is based upon symbolic communication an important question which demands attention concerns the range of images and vocabularies of ageing available to the members of any particular culture: just how many stories of ageing can we imagine? Just how many stories of ageing can we tell? Is, for example, the hope for a more positive substitution for what Gullette describes as the 'decline narrative' (1997) a realistic one so that at some point in the future ageing will no longer be the subject of stigma, fear, and disgust? And who will write these new stories? This question takes us into the future of ageing (the study of ageing in science fiction is a potentially rewarding field: see, for example, Hayles on 'The life cycle of cyborgs: writing the posthuman' (1999)); ageing of ethnic groups; and the search for evidence of changing attitudes towards ageing among members of younger age groups – anticipatory ageing: how do they see the future? The most important question concerns the future of ageing: do cultural developments and changes promise new opportunities and an expanding array of lifestyles as we grow older, or are there limitations on the oppor-tunities in the future (Blaikie 1999)?

These questions are crucial to the development of social gerontology in a rapidly changing world because they are absolutely central to the social constructionist argument that human meanings of ageing are socially created and thus malleable and open to future change. It still remains to be seen if evidence can be discovered in researching cultural products to show that this is the case, but the effort is potentially enriching.

Further reading

Ansello, E.F. (1977) Age and ageism in children's first literature, *Educational Geron-tology*, 2: 255–74.

Arnold, J.V. (1993) Montherlant and the problem of the ageing pederast, in A.M. Wyatt-Brown and J. Rossen (eds) *Ageing and Gender in Literature: Studies in Creativity*. Charlottesville, VA and London: University Press of Virginia.

Bradley, S. (1999) 'Visiting a war-zone': experiencing the ageing process in fiction. Unpub PhD, Department of Sociology, University of Aberdeen.

Charles, D.C. and Charles, L.A. (1979–80) Charles Dickens' old people, *International Journal of Ageing and Human Development*, 10(3): 231–7.

Cole, T.R., Van Tassel, D.D. and Kastenbaum, R. (eds) (1992) *Handbook of The Humanities and Ageing*. New York, NY: Springer Publishing Co.

Featherstone, M. and Wernick, A. (1995) *Images of Ageing: Cultural Representations of Later Life*. London and New York, NY: Routledge.

Harper, S. and Victor, C. (eds) (1997) *Critical Approaches to Ageing and Later Life*. Buckingham: Open University Press.

Hepworth, M. and Featherstone, M. (1982) *Surviving Middle Age*. Oxford: Basil Blackwell.

Holt, H. and Pym, H. (eds) (1984) *A Very Private Eye: The Diaries, Letters and Notebooks of Barbara Pym*. London: Macmillan.

Johnson, J. and Slater, R. (eds) (1993) *Ageing and Later Life*. London: Sage Publica-tions/The Open University.

Kenney, C. (1991) Detecting a novel use for spinsters in Sayers's fiction, in L.L. Doan (ed.) *Old Maids to Radical Spinsters: Unmarried Woman in The Twentieth-Century Novel*. Urbana and Chicago, IL: University of Illinois Press.

Lancet (1999) Literature and Ageing, Special Issue: Vol. 354, supplement 3, 6 November.

Lowenthal, D. (1985) *The Past is a Foreign Country*. Cambridge: Cambridge University Press.

Manthorpe, J. (1995) Private residential care in fiction, *Generations Review*, 5(1): 6.

Porter, L. and Porter, L.M. (eds) (1984) *Ageing in Literature*. Troy, NY: International.

Sohngen, M. (1975) The writer as an old woman, *The Gerontologist*, December: 493–8.

Sokoloff, J. (1987) *The Margin that Remains: A Study of Ageing in Literature*. New York, NY: Peter Lang.

Spicker, S.F., Woodward, K.M. and Van Tassel, D.D. (eds) (1978) *Ageing and The Elderly: Humanistic Perspectives in Gerontology*. Atlantic Highlands, NJ: Humanities Press Inc.

Woodward, K.M. (1991) *Ageing and its Discontents: Freud and Other Fictions*. Bloomington, IN: Indiana University Press.

Woodward, K.M. and Schwartz, M.M. (eds) (1986) *Memory and Desire: Ageing – Literature – Psychoanalysis*. Bloomington, IN: Indiana University Press.

Wyatt-Brown, A.M. and Rossen, J. (eds) (1993) *Ageing and Gender in Literature: Studies in Creativity*. Charlottesville, VA: University Press of Virginia.

Zeilig, H. (1997) The uses of literature in the study of older people, in A. Jamieson, S. Harper and C. Victor (eds) *Critical Approaches to Ageing and Later Life*. Buckingham: Open University Press.

References

Blaikie, A. (1999) *Ageing and Popular Culture*. Cambridge: Cambridge University Press.

Bond, J., Coleman, P. and Peace, S. (1993) *Ageing in Society: An Introduction to Social Gerontology*, second edn. London: Sage Publications.

Bytheway, B. (1995) *Ageism*. Buckingham: Open University Press.

Cole, T.R. and Gadow, S. (eds) (1986) *What Does it Mean to Grow Old? Reflections from the Humanities*. Durham: Duke University Press.

Cole, T.R. and Winkler, M.G. (eds) (1994) *The Oxford Book of Ageing*. Oxford: Oxford University Press.

Craig, P. and Cadogan, M. (1981) *The Lady Investigates: Women Detectives and Spies in Fiction*. London: Gollancz.

Freedman, R. (1978) Sufficiently decayed: gerontophobia in English literature, in S.F. Spicker, K.M. Woodward and D.D. Van Tassel (eds) *Ageing and the Elderly: Humanistic Perspectives in Gerontology*. Atlantic Highlands, NJ: Humanities Press.

Freeman, M. (1997) Death, narrative integrity, and the radical challenge of self-understanding: a reading of Tolstoy's *Death of Ivan Illych, Ageing and Society*, 17: 373–98.

Gullette, M.M. (1988) *Safe At Last in the Middle Years: The Invention of the Midlife Progress Novel: Saul Bellow, Margaret Drabble, Anne Tyler, and John Updike*. Berkeley, CA: University of California Press.

Gullette, M.M. (1997) *Declining to Decline: Cultural Combat and the Politics of the Midlife*. Charlottesville, VA and London: University Press of Virginia.

Hayles, N.K. (1999) The life cycle of cyborgs: writing the posthuman, in J. Wolmark (ed.) *Cybersexualities: A Reader on Feminist Theory, Cyborgs and Cyberspace*. Edinburgh: Edinburgh University Press.

Hepworth, M. (1993) Old age in crime fiction in J. Johnson and R. Slater (eds) *Ageing and Later Life*. London: Sage Publications/The Open University.

Hepworth, M. (1995) 'Wrinkles of vice and wrinkles of virtue': the moral interpretation of the ageing body, in C. Hummel and J. Lalive D'Eppinay (eds) *Images of Ageing in Western Societies*. Geneva: Centre For Interdisciplinary Gerontology, University of Geneva.

Hepworth, M. (1996) William and the old folks: notes on infantilisation, *Ageing and Society*, 16: 423–41.

Hepworth, M. (2000) *Stories of Ageing*. Buckingham: Open University Press.

Hepworth, M. (forthcoming) 'The changes and chances of this mortal life': aspects of ageing in the fiction of Stanley Middleton, *Ageing and Society*.

Hockey, J. and James, A. (1993) *Growing Up and Growing Old: Ageing and Dependency in the Life Course*. London: Sage.

Homans, M. and Munich, A. (eds) (1997) *Remaking Queen Victoria*. Cambridge: Cambridge University Press.

Humphrey, R. (1993) Life stories and social careers: ageing and social life in an ex-mining town, *Ageing and Society*, 27(1): 166–78.

Katz, S. (1996) *Disciplining Old Age: The Formation of Gerontological Knowledge*. Charlottesville, VA and London: University Press of Virginia.

Kehl, D.G. (1988) The distaff and the staff: stereotypes and archetypes of the older woman in representative modern literature, *International Journal of Ageing and Human Development*, 26(1): 1–12.

Manthorpe, J. (2000) Dementia in contemporary fiction and biography, *Journal of Dementia Care*, May/June: 35–7.

Nappo, S. (1998) *Pompeii: Guide to the Lost City*. London: Weidenfeld and Nicolson.

Rooke, C. (1992) Old age in contemporary fiction: a new paradigm of hope, in T.R. Cole, D.D. Van Tassel and R. Kastenbaum (eds) *Handbook of the Humanities and Ageing*. New York, NY: Springer Publishing Co.

Sarton, M. (1996) *At Eighty-Two: A Journal*. London: The Women's Press.

Shaw, M. and Vanacker, S. (1991) *Reflecting on Miss Marple*. London and New York, NY: Routledge.

Stewart, A. (1997) *Art, Desire and The Body in Ancient Greece*. Cambridge: Cambridge University Press.

Wyatt-Brown, A.M. (1989a) The narrative imperative: fiction and the ageing writer, *Journal of Ageing Studies*, 3(1): 55–65.

Wyatt-Brown, A.M. (1989b) Creativity in midlife: the novels of Anita Brookner, *Journal of Ageing Studies*, 3(2): 175–81.

Wyatt-Brown, A.M. (1992a) Literary gerontology comes of age, in T. Cole, D.D. Van Tassel and R. Kastenbaum (eds) *Handbook of the Humanities and Ageing*. New York, NY: Springer.

Wyatt-Brown, A.M. (1992b) *Barbara Pym: A Critical Biography*. Columbia, MO and London: University of Missouri Press.

Zeilig, H. (1999) Older people and their families in 1920s popular fiction: fictions of age and their importance for social gerontology. Unpublished PhD, University of London.

Novels cited

When there are two dates cited, the first is the date of first publication and the second the date of the copy consulted.

Bailey, P. ([1967] 1987) *At The Jerusalem*. London: Penguin.

Barker, P. (1986) *The Century's Daughter*. London: Virago.

Bawden, N. (1997; 1991) *Family Money*. London: Virago.

Conlon, K. ([1985] 1986) *Face Values*. London: Coronet.

Dexter, C. ([1989] 1990) *The Wench is Dead*. London: Pan.

Ewing, B. (1997) *The Actresses*. London: Little, Brown & Co.

Galsworthy, J. (1942) *The Forsyte Saga*. London: William Heinemann.

Gilbert, A. ([1946] 1987) *The Spinster's Secret*. London: Pandora.

Herriot, J. (1970) *If Only They Could Talk*. London: Pan.

Isler, A. ([1994] 1996) *The Prince of West End Avenue*. London: Vintage.

Laurence, M. ([1964] 1987) *The Stone Angel*. London: Virago.

Lee, L. (1962) *Cider with Rosie*. Harmondsworth: Penguin.

Middleton, S. (1991) *Beginning to End*. London: Hutchinson.

Pym, B. ([1977] 1994)*Quartet in Autumn*. London: Flamingo.

Robinson, P. ([1999] 2000) *In a Dry Season*. London: Pan.

Sackville-West, V. ([1931] 1989) *All Passion Spent*. London: Virago.

Sarton, M. ([1973] 1992) *As We Are Now*. London: The Women's Press.

Smiley, J. ([1981] 1995) *At Paradise Gate*. London: Flamingo.

Sutton, H. (1995) *Gorleston*. London: Sceptre.

Taylor, E. ([1971] 1996) *Mrs Palfrey at The Claremont*. London: Virago.

Walpole, H. (1927) *The Old Ladies*. London: Macmillan.

White, P. (1975) *The Eye of the Storm*. Harmondsworth: Penguin.

Part *III*

Creating new data

7

Doing longitudinal research
Michael Wadsworth

Introduction

Two markers of time passing have changed greatly over the last hundred years. First is the length of life. Second is the rate of change of society.

Life expectation became longer quickly in the twentieth century and the proportion of people who now live to be age 80 years and over has grown. Contemporary social change was a necessary part of that increase in life expectation (McKeown and Lowe 1966; Wilkinson 1996; Marmot and Wilkinson 1999), but has itself become so rapid that it is now the norm to experience considerable change during a lifetime in terms of technological factors, and in work and family life, behaviour, attitudes and expectations (Halsey and Webb 2000). These changes have far-reaching implications for the life course and the experience of later life.

New generations reaching later life are soon to differ considerably from our present image of that time in terms, for example, of vigour, income, interests, expectations, and geographical mobility, and in their experience of family life. In many respects these changes will be brought by the factors salient in bringing about the increase in life expectancy, namely improvement in nutrition; increasingly effective medical care and lay awareness of how to maintain health; greater opportunities in education and literacy; and greatly improved distributions of income and wealth, and conditions at work and at home (Marwick 1982; Halsey and Webb 2000).

Increasingly, notions of how ageing occurs are concerned with long-term effects, both intrinsic and extrinsic, and the interactions between them. In

health, for example, Forsdahl (1978) suggested that the rise in heart disease risk in the second half of the twentieth century was caused by overweight. He speculated that growing up in poverty and being an adult in
times of plenty was the basis of the problem. This seminal paper draws
attention to three of the most fundamental questions about ageing and
health. First, it raises the question of whether aspects of childhood as well
as adult life should be considered as part of the process of ageing. Second it
asks whether the interaction of child and adult factors might be one of the
ways in which the process operates. Third it indicates, implicitly, the changing
nature of risk, and the probability that risk exposure is likely to be unique
for each generation.

Since Forsdahl's paper a whole new theory of biological programming
has been developed (Reid 1969; Barker 1992, 1998), based on observations
of the relationship of growth in the prenatal period and in infancy to
health in adulthood. Poor growth in early life is associated with reduced
health chances throughout life. Biological thinking suggests that, because
most organ development is completed before birth or very shortly afterwards, that period of life should be regarded as a time of programming for
the rest of life (Barker 1998). This notion of biological programming does
not exclude the effect of risk and protective factors encountered at later
stages in life. For example, own smoking in adulthood is damaging to
health, and because the capacity of the respiratory system is fixed early in
life, the extent of that damage will be related to the respiratory capacity
established early in life. So biological programming can be seen as the
development of health capital for the rest of life. The implications of this,
and of Forsdahl's work, are that the historical time of early life will leave its
imprint on each generation, since most aspects of health and growth in
early life are powerfully influenced by their socioeconomic context
(Wadsworth 1991). There are comparable social science theories that assert
that the social context of childhood and adolescence is associated with the
context of adult life. For example, strong associations are found between
educational opportunity and adult socioeconomic circumstances (Douglas
1964; Wadsworth 1991; Kuh *et al.* 1997), and between the early development of temperamental and behavioural style and adult behaviour (Caspi
and Moffitt 1993; Elder *et al.* 1993). There is increasing evidence that the
basis for the individual's biological and social capital is laid down before
adult life, and thereafter the interaction of the capital with the circumstances of adulthood determines many important aspects of life and life
chances.

The implications of these ideas for the population in later life are profound, particularly in a rapidly changing social context. Improvements in
child health prefigure a generation that will carry that benefit throughout
life, and probably into old age, although a generation carrying the big
postwar changes in that benefit has yet to reach later life. Widening opportunities in education, which first began in the cohorts born towards the

end the Second World War, will bring generations that differ in later life from their predecessors in skills, health, wealth, expectations and demands. The benefits of twentieth-century improvements in health can already be seen in the increased longevity of the British population. So far that increase is largely the result of improvements in the health of adults, as medical care came to be more effective from the 1950s onwards. The effect of improvements in the health of children will be seen first in the postwar baby boom cohort as it arrives at later life.

The likelihood of a longer later life has changed views about later life, and stimulated concern about how to keep the population at that stage as healthy as possible. The population of that age used to be seen as comprising a hardy breed that had survived the earlier historical periods of highly prevalent poverty and infectious illness, and that had reached the time of life when a natural slowing down of functions was inevitable. When those views prevailed then interest in health in later life was low. Now that the proportion of those in later life is rising, the care of health at that stage has become of great concern, in terms of its cost and the need for preventive and therapeutic care, rather than simple maintenance of a tolerable level of function. The goal is to compress the period of debilitating illness and impairment as far as possible into a period at the end of life, rather than have it blight a longer period of later life. The next generation to arrive at the threshold of later life will demand better physical and cognitive functioning and better health than its predecessor generations.

These ideas about biological programming and its implications for later life have been developed and tested with the aid of longitudinal data on the life course. Such data are, however, in short supply because of the intrinsic difficulties in their collection (Kuh and Ben Shlomo 1997). The search for sources of information about the life course has produced innovative methods for looking at long periods of life. These collectively may be called longitudinal methods, and if they involve data collection that predates the outcome of interest they are also prospective. That period of predating need not necessarily be long, nor does the outcome of interest necessarily have to be defined at the beginning of the study for an investigation to have the advantages of this method.

The first characteristic advantage of the longitudinal method is that the sequence and chronology of events are known for the period of prospective data collection. This is a unique advantage that allows the researcher more than in any other method to comment on possible cause and effect relationships. The second characteristic is that although recall is required, with its commensurate risks of memory error and distortion, that period is usually only as long as the time elapsed since the previous data collection. The third feature of the prospective method is that it captures those kinds of information that can only be caught with accuracy contemporaneously, such as attitudes, biological and anthropological measures, and details of relationships and interactions between the social and physical environment. The fourth characteristic, particularly relevant in studies of health and ageing, is that a longitudinal study, if it starts in middle life or earlier, has a good chance of including those most at risk of premature death as compared with a study of ageing that begins in later life.

The aim of this chapter is to outline ways in which the longitudinal method has been used in studies of ageing, and to note some salient advantages and disadvantages of the methods. The emphasis is largely on health because that is where most innovative work on the study of individuals has been undertaken. Most examples are of large studies, but nothing in the definition of a longitudinal study requires it to be large. In this chapter the different concepts of time passing are discussed, because they have to be understood and managed in investigations that cover long periods. Then two methods of longitudinal data collection are described: those that cut short the period of waiting that is involved in a follow-up study, which are called here accelerated methods, and those that do not. The latter are described as wholly prospective methods. A long-term follow-up study is used to illustrate the benefits as well as the problems associated with the wholly prospective method.

The concept of time passing

Time passes for society in the sense of historical time, and for the individual in the sense of growth, development and ageing. When historical time and the individual experience of time are considered together it is necessary to differentiate age, cohort and period effect.

Age effects

The individual's experience of time passing is known as an age effect. It can be described in terms of development and ageing. An age effect impacts at or about a specific age, regardless of historical time; menarche and the menopause are examples of age effects.

Cohort effects

Cohort effects are those that impact on one age group or cohort in the population. For instance, the rise in women smoking in the years before the Second World War is a cohort effect, particularly as it mostly affected women in early adulthood (Todd 1975). Those exposed to a particular drug (e.g.diethylstilbestrol) that was for a time prescribed during pregnancy, and

Table 7.1 Life expectation at birth and at age 40 years in populations corresponding to the 1946 cohort population, their parents' generation and their children's generation

| | Years of birth of | | | | |
| | Parents' generation | | Own generation | Children's generation | |
	1901	1931	1951[a]	1971	1981
Expectation of years of life at birth in each year					
Males	48	58	66	67	70
Females	52	62	72	75	76
Expectation of age at death among those born in the given year and surviving to age 40 years					
Males	67	69	71	72	72
Females	69	72	75	77	78
Gains in expectation of years more life after age 40 years compared with expectation at birth					
Males	19	11	5	5	2
Females	17	10	3	2	2

[a] Year nearest to 1946 for which national data are available

which is now regarded as a possible long-term risk for cancer, are a cohort with that specific risk exposure (Holford 1991).

Period effects

A period effect impacts on everyone at a particular time. For example, food rationing during the Second World War and the immediate postwar years affected the whole population. The impact of the peaks of atmospheric pollution in London in the 1950s also affected the whole population, and caused an increased risk in the vulnerable of any age (Holland *et al.* 1979). During the twentieth century, education, occupation and unemployment, nutrition, smoking, the distribution of wealth and purchasing power and the role of women in society have all differed with generation (Holford 1991; Halsey and Webb 2000). This is particularly evident in expectation of years of life where changes in the circumstances of both childhood and adult life have brought considerable inter- and intragenerational difference (Table 7.1).

Accelerated prospective designs

The catch-up design

In the catch-up design, a population that has already been the subject of study at an earlier time is identified for further study at a later time, usually but not necessarily through records. There is, for instance, a later life follow-up of survivors of the famine inflicted on a province in the Netherlands by Nazi occupying forces during the Second World War. During the famine obstetric hospitals continued to keep records of their patients' health, and these have been used to show the effect of meagre and deficient maternal diet on the developing foetus. A catch-up study of adults born during that period showed correlations between stage in pregnancy at which poor maternal nutrition occurred and subsequent health in the early developmental years and later adult life (Susser and Stein 1994).

In Britain catch-up design studies were used to collect data that led to the concept of biological programming. That work used detailed birth records that were found for the period 1911–30. The individuals who were the subjects of the records were traced in later adult life (in the late 1980s and early 1990s), and their blood pressure and respiratory function were measured, in order to explore the hypothesis that the evidence of prenatal growth provided by the birth records would be associated with the adult outcome measures (Barker 1992, 1998). The catch-up design was also used to study the relationship of childhood nutrition on health and survival in later life in the Boyd-Orr study. A study of family diet and health had been undertaken in 1937 and 1939, in which 1352 families kept records of food bought and eaten, details of socioeconomic circumstances were reported, and measures were made of the children's growth (Gunnell *et al.* 1996). A follow-up of mortality records of child participants in this study was used to show the association of poor living conditions and diet in childhood with an increased risk of coronary heart disease and possibly cancer in adulthood (Gunnell *et al.* 1998).

In the USA death certificates of a sample of high-IQ Californian children first studied in a longitudinal investigation that began in 1921 have been followed up for research into longevity and causes of death, in relation to a number of factors such as personality, adult psychological adjustment, and changes in marital status and in the family of origin and own generation, and smoking (Friedman *et al.* 1995; Tucker *et al.* 1997). Those studies concluded that psychosocial factors and the experience of parental separation during childhood were associated with the raised risk of premature death. The US Berkeley Guidance and Oakland Growth Studies have also been fertile sources of results from their follow-up studies conducted after the populations of the initial investigations during childhood were identified in adult life. These studies have been concerned with the effects of economic deprivation experienced during the Depression years on adult behaviour and socioeconomic outcomes, which included parental behaviour and its apparent effects across generations. These long-term studies showed how adverse and stressful experience tended to exaggerate or develop behaviour traits and characteristics that already exist, thus providing evidence about the interaction of the social environment with individual attributes (Caspi and Elder 1988; Caspi and Moffitt 1993; Elder *et al.* 1993). These and other US studies are described in Giele and Elder (1998).

Strengths of the catch-up method are that it does not rely on recall for many aspects of data collection; there is no element of waiting for time to pass and for individuals to age, because that has already happened; and the chronological order of events is likely to be known with much greater precision than in other data collection methods that do not have a longitudinal element.

Weaknesses are that neither the population selected nor the data collected in the original study may be entirely what the new researcher wants, and the population available will be survivors, which for some purposes may limit what can be done. Nevertheless, as the Boyd-Orr follow-up of health in later life showed, even the non-survivor population may provide information, in the case of cause of death and age at death (Gunnell *et al.* 1998).

The mixed catch-up and prospective design

These studies usually begin in adulthood, and use recall methods to collect information about the past, as well as prospective follow-up methods. For example, the new English National Study of Ageing takes as its population a large sample of men and women aged 50 years and over who were respondents in two of the annual representative samples of the national health surveys (Erens and Primatesta 1999). Data from the original health surveys will provide baseline information about midlife social circumstances and health, and follow up will be concerned with health, cognition and socioeconomic circumstances. Data on health, development and socioeconomic circumstances in childhood, and on earlier adult life health and circumstances, will be collected using recall methods. This study will be multidimensional, and valuable not only for its health content, but also because of its wide range of economic data as well as information on social and family networks and support and their change with retirement and with increasing age.

The Bonn Longitudinal Study of Ageing is of a similar design (Rudinger and Thomae 1990). It is concerned with the cognitive theory of personality, based on the subjects' experience of learning and of social circumstances earlier in life, which was established by recollection methods. These were related to measures of satisfaction and psychological well-being, and to such objective indicators as income, education and physician-assessed health. Of similar design, rather more concentrated on physical health, are the Duke Longitudinal Studies of Ageing (Palmore *et al.* 1985), Svanborg's (1988) studies of Swedish cohorts, and the Berlin Study of Ageing (Smith and Baltes 1993). Baltes and Baltes (1990), Giele and Elder (1998) and the European Commission (1999) review a number of comparable longitudinal studies.

An ingenious-cross cohort element has been added to the mixed catch-up and prospective designs in a study of the health of three cohorts of Glasgow residents (MacIntyre *et al.* 1989). The cohorts were aged 15, 35 and 55 years at the beginning of the study, and each cohort has given retrospective information, and has been followed up at later ages. This provides an element of generational comparison in addition to the use of the mixed method.

The *strengths* of this mixed catch-up and prospective method for studies of ageing are that it allows the researcher to select the population for study; there need be no very long wait for ageing to take place; the prospective data collection provides the opportunity to collect whatever information and measures are desired in order to measure age-related change; and the chronological order of events is likely to be correct.

The *weakness* of this method for some purposes lies in the reliance on recall for information about earlier times in life, and in the fact that the population, by definition, comprises survivors.

The wholly prospective design

Britain has five substantial birth cohort studies. The first, known as the MRC National Survey of Health and Development (NSHD), began in 1946 with a population of 5362 first studied at birth (Wadsworth 1991). The second, known as the National Child Development Study (NCDS) or the 1958 British Birth Cohort Study, began in 1958 also at birth and with a population of 17,414 (Ferri 1993). The third, which was known as Child Health and Education in the Seventies (CHES), but is now usually referred to as the 1970 British Birth Cohort Study, began at birth in 1970 with a population of 17,198 (Bynner *et al.* 1997). The fourth began in 1991/92 during the mother's pregnancy, and that is known as the Avon Longitudinal Study of Pregnancy and Childbirth (ALSPAC), with a population of 14,000 (Golding *et al.* 2001). The most recent national birth cohort, known as the Millennium Birth Cohort Study, began in 2000 with a population of 12,000 and a first data collection at age 8 months. The 1946, 1958, 1970 and 2000 studies are nationally representative, and the 1984 cohort is of births in the Avon area. The most recent data collection in the 1946 study was at age 55 years (1999), in the 1958 cohort at 42 years (2000), in the 1970 study at 30 years (2000), in the 1991/92 study at 8 years, and in the 2000 cohort the most recent contact was the first.

Funding for such studies is ideally by programme grant to maintain the core team that designs the data collections, maintains the archive of data and the contact details for the study population, and undertakes most analysis. Funding for data collections and for some analyses is often obtained from specialist funding agencies.

The focus of topics of research in such large-scale investigations is inevitably policy-related. Each study was concerned particularly with health in the early years of its cohort's lives, and with education, behaviour and health during the school years. This has provided rich sources of information on growth and mental and physical development, and the family and social contexts in the years before adulthood. That information is used now for the study of pathways from childhood to adult outcomes. For example, those studies have shown the relevance of infant school experience and parents' interest in education as markers of likely educational attainment (Douglas 1964; Fogelman 1983), and the importance of growth in early life to such indicators of ageing as blood pressure in childhood and adult life (Wadsworth *et al.* 1985; Whincup *et al.* 1999), cognitive function (Richards *et al.* 2001), and midlife obesity (Hardy *et al.* 2000; Kuh *et al.* in press). Early growth has also been found to be a raised risk for breast cancer (De Stavola *et al.* 2000). These studies have also explored risks to educational attainment and to midlife physical and mental health associated with the childhood experience of parental separation (Rodgers 1994; Richards *et al.* 1997; Ely *et al.* 1999); the long-term adverse effects on health and well-being of poor socioeconomic circumstances, particularly in early life (Power *et al.* 1991, 1996; Baker *et al.* 1998; Wadsworth *et al.* in press); and the long-term effects of prolonged unemployment (Montgomery *et al.* 1998; Wadsworth *et al.* 1999).

Each of these studies has unprecedented data on development, and the three whose populations are already adult are providing unique data for research into the processes of ageing. I will now use the oldest study to illustrate the value of these resources, and the difficulties in carrying out such studies, as well as benefits.

Case study: *The 1946 birth cohort study*

The sample

A permanent feature that is usually selected only once at the beginning of a prospective study is the population sample. This involves particularly difficult decisions if the study is intended to be, or becomes, a long-term investigation. A good estimate must be made of what the sample loss will be throughout the life of the study, from all causes, that is including death, refusal and migration, because the sample size must remain sufficient, after these losses, for all future purposes, in terms of statistical power and representativeness. The longer the time period proposed, and the greater the number of measures, the larger the population size required.

The original sample for the study of birth in the 1946 cohort comprised all the births (n = 16,687) that took place in England, Wales and Scotland in one week in March 1946 (Wadsworth 1991; Wadsworth *et al.* 1991). For the follow-up study sampling was necessary to reduce the population size in order to reduce costs, and to keep within limits set by the contemporary information technology. The sample was chosen to preserve the national representation, and to give similar numbers in each social class. That was achieved by selecting one in four of all babies born to wives of non-manual and agricultural workers, and all babies born to wives of manual workers. Babies born illegitimately were excluded because most were then adopted, and therefore could not be traced for follow-up. Twins and other multiple births were excluded because the numbers were thought too small for analysis.

In the long run the sample design of the 1946 study has offered the *advantages* that

- loss from moving is restricted to migration from the country because the whole country is included;
- the population size is small enough to make frequent data collections possible. This study carried out 11 data collections in the pre-school and school years and 10 data collections in the adult years up to age 43 years. In comparison the two subsequent cohorts which followed up all the births from the chosen week each had only four data collections during the pre-school and school years; thereafter up to 42 years the 1958 study has made three collections, and up to age 30 years the 1970 made two collections.

The sample design of the 1946 study has the *disadvantages* that

- numbers are small for the study of some events (e.g. there are 50 people with diabetes and 35 with schizophrenia), but studies have still been possible (Jones *et al.* 1994);
- numbers are too small for the study of rare events such as multiple sclerosis (one case).

Data collection methods

In the 1946 birth cohort health visitors, teachers, school health staff, and youth employment officers collected data during the pre-school and school years, using a wide range of instruments and methods, including cognitive tests (verbal, non-verbal and numerical), personality and behaviour ratings, questionnaires to mothers and teachers, and assessments made by health

and education staff (Wadsworth 1991). In adulthood postal questionnaires have been used and professional interviewers have made home
visits for data collections. Research nurses have also made home visits, at
the most recent, for example, to measure height, weight, blood pressure,
respiratory and cognitive function, balance and grip strength, to examine
knees and hands for early signs of osteoarthritis, and to ask a range of
questions about health and socioeconomic and family circumstances. On
three occasions in adulthood cohort members were asked to keep diet
diaries (Price *et al.* 1995). The study team twice recruited and trained nurses
and data collection has twice been contracted to the National Centre for
Social Research.

The impact of period effects

All aspects of the scientific work of longitudinal studies are influenced by
period effect, from the initial formulation of aims to the interpretation of
findings. For instance, questions about policy are inevitably those of the
present. Thus the concern with education policy in the 1946 study was
with the 'the waste of talent' that was perceived in the 1950s and 1960s in
numbers of children with high IQ who did not go into higher education
(Douglas 1964).

Period effect also touches the choice of measures at each data collection.
This may be because at some point data collections have preceded new
knowledge. For example, information about smoking by parents or children was not collected during the cohort's pre-school and school years
because the first papers showing the apparently harmful effects were not
published until the 1950s. It can also be because measurement techniques
were not at that time developed sufficiently, if at all. An example of that is
seen in the development of the Rutter Malaise Scale, which has been used
in the 1958 and 1970 cohorts, but was not developed in time for use in the
1946 cohort. The latter study had to use teachers' assessments of behaviour
rather than the more reliable Rutter Scale (Rutter 1967). A third type of
effect is that of change in measurement instrumentation. In the adult life
of this population blood pressure measuring equipment first used has
become obsolete. Period effect applies also to coding methods. Systems of
classification of occupations and diseases are developed and change over
time, so that in a prospective study data classified at the time of collection
may need to be reclassified with the more up-to-date systems in order to
maintain comparability with other studies. Period effects apply to ethical
considerations too. At the beginning of this study there was no necessity,
as there is now, for each participant to give informed consent.

Such inescapable effects of historical period are also a problem when
deciding how best to design a new data collection to be as relevant as
possible for future needs. So in the cohort's middle life it has been possible

only to use current ideas about aetiological pathways to risk of ill health in later life. In order to maximize the likelihood that data collected in middle life will be appropriate for future questions about how risk developed and was reduced, it is necessary not only to have the best advice about current hypotheses, but also to measure, code and store data in the finest detail possible. It would be wrong, for example, to code and store dietary data only in terms of particular micronutrients currently thought to be of greatest relevance to health in later life (e.g. vitamin C, calcium). In practice dietary data has to be kept on the broadest possible spectrum of detail (Prynne *et al.* 1999).

Nevertheless, despite its limitations and restrictions, period effect is also of considerable value. In times of rapid social change a study of the developing individual provides opportunities to test hypotheses about how the social environment has its impact. The population of the 1946 study lived through periods of greatly differing advice about such health-related behaviour and custom as smoking, diet, exercise and alcohol consumption. By observing how individuals reacted to that changing advice it has been possible to develop new ideas about how individual attributes and styles of presentation of self interact with current custom in a way that is strongly associated with health-related behaviour (Schooling 2001).

In summary the *advantage* of period effect in wholly prospective longitudinal studies is that

- in a long-term study the effects of changes in the social environment can be identified and their effects studied as the population ages; that advantage is greater in Britain where the opportunity exists to compare findings across the national birth cohorts in order to investigate the effects of differences in the social context at the same age.

The *disadvantage* of period effect in longitudinal studies is that

- data collections, coding methods and all aspects of the study can only be informed by the science of their time.

Topics studied in the 1946 birth cohort study

The broad concern of the 1946 study has always been with age-related health change. In childhood and adolescence this took the form of physical and mental development, and in adult life it is the processes of ageing. Fortunately this broadly defined concern has been maintained within the specific projects required to support the study. So, for example, information on mental development was collected using cognitive tests at ages 8, 11, and 15 years. Test scores were used to show the efficacy of contemporary education policy that aimed to identify, by examination at age 11 years, the highest scoring children for preparation for further and higher education. These results have also been of unique value since, as a source for showing the early life precursors of cognitive function (Richards *et al.* 2001), and for showing the relationship of childhood cognitive function with midlife memory (Richards *et al.* 1999).

In adult life the study's concern with health and its change with age has been guided by the opportunity to explore models of ageing processes in relation to the concept of biological programming, and the concept of ageing as the product of the accumulation of risk and protective factors throughout life. Each of these models is studied in relation to the social and scientific context, and is informed by new thinking about why and how social circumstances can precipitate ill health and influence health-related behaviour (Brunner 2000; Schooling 2001). Three types of markers of ageing are used. They are measures of function (e.g. respiratory function, blood pressure, cognitive function), measures of illness experienced, and measures of impairment. Selection of indicators of ageing has been governed so far by four factors: new measures have to be compatible with those used at earlier ages; they have to be age-appropriate; they must be usable as a baseline against which to measure future change; and they must be usable by research nurses at home visits.

Measures have so far been confined to those that can be made by research nurses at home visits, in order to maintain the study's high response rates (Wadsworth *et al.* 1991).

The value of the 1946 birth cohort as a source of information about ageing

The study's data have unique value for testing models of the effects of earlier life factors on later life. Having data collected throughout life provides the opportunity to examine the powerful effect of the interaction of childhood and adult factors. For instance, poor home circumstances in childhood are thought to be a long-term risk to health, arguably because such circumstances are conducive neither to optimum growth nor to good educational attainment, and poor growth and low educational attainment are associated with risk to adult health. Table 7.2 shows that men and women who experienced poor home circumstances in infancy, and who were in the lowest third of weight at birth and of height at age 2 years, were at increased risk of having raised blood pressure at age 43 years. This effect was seen in those who at 43 years were neither overweight nor obese, and it was greatly increased in those who were overweight or obese. This shows that the early life effects are not inescapably deterministic. Clearly by no means all those with adverse growth and early life circumstances had this health problem by 43 years. And clearly avoiding being

Table 7.2 Infant social circumstances, prenatal and postnatal growth in relation to body mass index (weight/height) and raised blood pressure at age 43 years (% with systolic bp = 140 mmHg or treated)

Aggregate score of father's social class, infant crowding,* birth weight,** height** at 2 yrs	Body mass index at age 43 years	
	Not overweight nor obese***	Overweight or obese
Men	(n = 585)	(n = 661)
Best score	13.1%	12.2%
	14.0%	19.2%
Worst score	15.9%	29.1%
	(NS)	(p < 0.001)
Women	(n = 715)	(n = 435)
Best score	8.0%	8.0%
	9.7%	15.9%
Worst score	17.2%	24.1%
	(p = 0.02)	(p < 0.001)

* 2 or more persons per room
** in equal thirds
*** BMI < 25

overweight or obese in adulthood is associated with a reduction in the risk that is carried from childhood.

The *value* of the 1946 cohort to studies of ageing may be summarized as follows:

- it indicates the nature and extent of functional change with age in a representative population;
- it provides opportunities to determine pathways, both in terms of risk and prevention, from earlier life to later outcomes;
- it allows evaluation of the predictive power of experiences, events and health to affect later life;
- it has the ability to show the likely state of health on arrival at the threshold of later life of the generation now in middle life, and how it will in that respect differ from its predecessor generation;
- it offers the opportunity of comparisons with later born generations studied in the other large birth cohort studies and therefore the evaluation of different kinds of period and cohort effects.

Conclusions

The demand for longitudinal data covering long periods of the life course has produced a range of resources, and ingenious methods for their exploitation, in the study of ageing and the effects on ageing of interactions of biological and psychological factors and the social environment.

Studies that use longitudinal information show how the social, behavioural and biological characteristics of people differ in each generation, and show that the later life of generations now in middle and early adulthood will be different from that of any earlier generation. Through the study of developmental processes and experiences in the years before later life begins, it is increasingly possible to anticipate some important features of the later life of future generations.

Such studies also provide information about how individuals age during the life course. A comprehensive and encouraging framework within which constructive discussion about new research into current and future patterns of human ageing can take place is offered by Baltes and Baltes (1990) in their demonstration of resilience in later life. Opportunities exist in long-term prospective studies to investigate precursors of resilience.

In future, studies of ageing will have increasingly rich sources of longitudinal data. In Britain the four national birth cohorts and the comprehensive study of children in Avon offer the opportunity to compare prospectively collected life course data on representative samples born at different social, economic and cultural times. Other European countries, particularly Finland, offer similar longitudinal investigations, and a wide range of studies of ageing (European Commission 1999).

An important feature of the new interest in life course research has been the discovery of past studies on which to capitalize, in order to gain immediately the view of a long stretch of time, or of the individual life course. Many more opportunities to do that await the investigator in the many existing follow-up studies of education, social mobility, employment and unemployment, and in the intervention studies in health.

References

Baker, D., Taylor, H., Henderson, J. and ALSPAC Team (1998) Inequality in infant morbidity, *Journal of Epidemiology and Mental Health*, 52: 451–8.

Baltes, P.B. and Baltes, M.M. (1990) *Successful Aging*. New York, NY: Cambridge University Press.

Barker, D.J.P. (1992) *Fetal and Infant Origins of Adult Disease*. London: BMJ Publishing.

Barker, D.J.P. (1998) *Mothers and Babies and Health in Later Life*, 2nd edn. Edinburgh: Churchill Livingstone.

Brunner, E.J. (2000) Toward a new social biology, in L.F. Berkman and I. Kawachi (eds) *Social Epidemiology*. New York, NY: Oxford University Press.

Bynner, J., Ferri, E. and Shepherd, P. (eds) (1997) *Twenty-Something in the 1990s*. Aldershot: Dartmouth Press.

Caspi, A. and Elder, G.H. (1988) Emergent family patterns, in R.A. Hinde and J. Stevenson-Hinde (eds) *Relationships within Families*. New York, NY: Oxford University Press.

Caspi, A. and Moffitt, T.E. (1993) When do individual differences matter? *Psychological Inquiry*, 4: 247–71.

De Stavola, B.L., Hardy, R., Kuh, D. *et al.* (2000) Birth weight, childhood growth and risk of breast cancer in a British cohort, *British Journal of Cancer*, 83: 964–8.

Douglas, J.W.B. (1964) *The Home and the School*. London: McGibbon and Kee.

Elder, G.H., Modell, J. and Parke, R.E. (eds) (1993) *Children in Time and Place*. Cambridge: Cambridge University Press.

Ely, M., Richards, M.P.M., Wadsworth, M.E.J. and Elliott, B.J. (1999) Secular changes in the association of parental divorce and children's educational attainment: evidence from three British birth cohorts, *Journal of Social Policy*, 28: 437–55.

Erens, R. and Primatesta, P. (eds) (1999) *Cardiovascular Disease '98*. London: The Stationery Office.

European Commission (1999) *Survey on the Current Status of Research into 'Ageing' in Europe*. Luxembourg: Office for Official Publications of the European Communities.

Ferri, E. (ed.) (1993) *Life at 33: The Fifth Follow-up of the National Child Development Study*. London: National Children's Bureau.

Fogelman, K. (ed.) (1983) *Growing Up in Great Britain*. London: Macmillan.

Forsdahl, A. (1978) Living conditions in childhood and subsequent development of risk factors for arteriosclerotic heart disease, *Journal of Epidemiology and Public Health*, 32: 34–7.

Friedman, H.S., Tucker, J.S., Schwartz, J.E. *et al.* (1995) Psychosocial and behavioral predictors of longevity, *American Psychologist*, 50: 69–78.

Giele, J.Z. and Elder Jr, G.H. (1998) *Methods of Life Course Research: Qualitative and Quantitative Approaches*. Thousand Oaks, CA: Sage Publications.

Golding, J., Pembrey, M., Jones, R. and ALSPAC Study Team (2001) ALSPAC – the Avon Longitudinal Study of Parents and Children. 1: Study methodology, *Paediatric and Perinatal Epidemiology*, 15: 74–87.

Gunnell, D.J., Frankel, S., Nanchalal, K., Braddon, F.E.M. and Davey Smith, G. (1996) Life course and later disease: a follow-up study based on a survey of family diet and health in pre-war Britain (1937–9), *Public Health*, 110: 85–94.

Gunnell, D.J., Davey Smith, G., Frankel, S. *et al.* (1998) Childhood leg length and adult mortality: follow-up of the Carnegie (Boyd-Orr) survey of diet and health in pre-war Britain, *Journal of Epidemiology and Community Health*, 52: 142–52.

Halsey, A.H. and Webb, J. (2000) *Twentieth Century British Social Trends*. London: Macmillan.

Hardy, R., Wadsworth, M. and Kuh, D. (2000) The influence of childhood weight and socioeconomic status on change in adult body mass index in a British national birth cohort, *International Journal of Obesity*, 24: 725–34.

Holford, T.R. (1991) Understanding the effects of age, period and cohort on incidence and mortality rates, *Annual Review of Public Health*, 12: 425–57.

Holland, W.W., Bennett, A.E., Cameron, I.R. *et al.* (1979) Health effects of particulate pollution: reappraising the evidence, *American Journal of Epidemiology*, 110: 527–659.

Jones, P., Rodgers, B., Murray, R. and Marmot, M.G. (1994) Child developmental risk factors for adult schizophrenia in the British 1946 birth cohort, *Lancet*, 344: 1398–1402.

Kuh, D.J.L. and Ben Shlomo, Y. (eds) (1997) *A Life Course Approach to Chronic Disease Epidemiology*. Oxford: Oxford University Press.

Kuh, D.J.L., Head, J., Hardy, R.J. and Wadsworth, M.E.J. (1997) The influence of education and family background on women's earnings in midlife, *British Journal of the Sociology of Education*, 18: 385–405.

Kuh, D.J., Hardy, R., Chaturvedi, N. and Wadsworth, M. (in press) Birth weight, childhood growth and abdominal obesity in adult life, *International Journal of Obesity*.

MacIntyre, S., Annandale, E., Ecob, R. *et al.* (1989) The West of Scotland 2007 study of health in the community, in C. Martin and D. Macqueen (eds) *Readings for a New Public Health*, pp. 56–75. Edinburgh: Edinburgh University Press.

McKeown, T. and Lowe, C.R. (1966) *An Introduction to Social Medicine*. Oxford: Blackwell.

Marmot, M.G. and Wilkinson, R.J. (eds) (1999) *Social Determinants of Health*. Oxford: Oxford University Press.

Marwick, A. (1982) *British Society since 1940*. London: Penguin.

Montgomery, S.M., Cook, D.G., Bartley, M.J. and Wadsworth, M.E.J. (1998) Unemployment, cigarette smoking, alcohol consumption and body weight in young men, *European Journal of Public Health*, 8: 21–7.

Palmore, E., Busse, E.W., Maddox, G.L., Nowlin, J.B. and Siegler, I.C. (eds) (1985) *Normal Aging III: Reports from the Duke Longitudinal Studies, 1975–1984*. Durham: Duke University Press.

Power, C., Manor, O. and Fox, A.J. (1991) *Health and Class: The Early Years*. London: Chapman and Hall.

Power, C., Bartley, M., Davey Smith, G. and Blane, D. (1996) Transmission of social and biological risk across the life course, in D. Blane, E. Brunner and R.Wilkinson (eds) *Health and Social Organisation*, pp. 188–203. London: Routledge.

Price, G.M., Paul, A.A., Key, F.B. *et al.* (1995) Measurement of diet in a large national survey, *Journal of Human Nutrition and Dietetics*, 8: 417–28.

Prynne, C.J., Paul, A.A., Price, G.M. *et al.* (1999) Food and nutrient intake of a national sample of four year old children in 1950: comparison with the 1990s, *Public Health Nutrition*, 2: 537–47.

Reid, D.D. (1969) The beginnings of chronic bronchitis, *Proceedings of the Royal Society of Medicine*, 62: 311–16.

Richards, M., Hardy, R. and Wadsworth, M. (1997) The effects of divorce and separation on mental health in a national UK birth cohort, *Psychological Medicine*, 27: 1121–8.

Richards, M., Kuh, D.J.L., Hardy, R. and Wadsworth, M.E.J. (1999) Lifetime cognitive function and timing of the natural menopause, *Neurology*, 53: 308–14.

Richards, M., Hardy, R.J., Kuh, D.J.L. and Wadsworth, M.E.J. (2001) Birth weight and cognitive function in the British 1946 birth cohort, *British Medical Journal*, 322: 199–203.

Rodgers, B. (1994) Pathways between parental divorce and adult depression, *Journal of Child Psychology and Psychiatry*, 35: 1289–308.

Rudinger, G. and Thomae, H. (1990) The Bonn Longitudinal Study of Aging: coping, life adjustment, and life satisfaction, in P.B. Baltes and M.M. Baltes (eds) *Successful Aging*. New York, NY: Cambridge University Press.

Rutter, M. (1967) A children's behaviour questionnaire for completion by teachers, *Journal of Child Psychology and Psychiatry*, 9: 1–11.

Schooling, C.M. (2001) Health related behaviour in a social and temporal context. PhD thesis, University of London.

Smith, J. and Baltes, P.B. (1993) Differential psychological aging: profiles of the old and very old, *Ageing and Society*, 13: 551–87.

Susser, M. and Stein, Z. (1994) Timing in prenatal nutrition: a reprise of the Dutch famine study, *Nutrition Reviews*, 52: 84–94.

Svanborg, A. (1988) The health of the elderly population: results from longitudinal studies age-cohort comparisons, *Ciba Foundation Symposium 1988*, 134: 3–11.

Todd, G.F. (1975) *Changes in Smoking Habits in the UK*. London: Tobacco Research Council.

Tucker, J.S., Friedman, H.S., Schwartz, J.E. *et al.* (1997) Parental divorce: effects on individual behaviour and longevity, *Journal of Personality and Social Psychology*, 73: 381–91.

Wadsworth, M.E.J. (1991) *The Imprint of Time*. Oxford: Oxford University Press.

Wadsworth, M.E.J., Cripps, H.A., Midwinter, R.A. and Colley, J.R.T. (1985) Blood pressure at age 36 years and social and familial factors, cigarette smoking and body mass in a national birth cohort, *British Medical Journal*, 291: 1534–8.

Wadsworth, M.E.J., Mann, S.L., Rodgers, B. *et al.* (1991) Loss and representativeness in a 43 year follow-up of a national birth cohort, *Journal of Epidemiology and Community Health*, 46: 300–4.

Wadsworth, M.E.J., Montgomery, S.M. and Bartley, M.J. (1999) The persisting effect of unemployment on health and social well-being in men early in working life, *Social Science and Medicine*, 48: 1491–9.

Wadsworth, M.E.J., Hardy, R.J., Paul, A.A., Marshall, S.F. and Cole, T.J. (in press) Leg and trunk length at 43 years in relation to childhood health, diet and family circumstances; evidence from the 1946 national birth cohort, *International Journal of Epidemiology*.

Whincup, P.H., Bredow, M., Payne, F., Sadler, S., Golding, J. and ALSPAC Study Team (1999) Size at birth and blood pressure at 3 years of age: the Avon Longitudinal Study of Pregnancy and Childhod, *American Journal of Epidemiology*, 149: 730–9.

Wilkinson, R.G. (1996) *Unhealthy Societies: The Afflictions of Inequality*. London: Routledge.

8

Doing life history research
Joanna Bornat

Introduction

A life history approach brings many different yet interconnected rewards for the researcher with an interest in ageing. The story of an individual life told in the first person yields information about a generation and a cohort as well as accounts which are gendered, cultural and historical. It may throw light on forgotten or hidden aspects of past experience, bringing to the foreground lives which have been marginalized, disregarded and downgraded. It may challenge existing assumptions and dominant narratives with subversive evidence. Perhaps most rewarding for the gerontologist, as a process it has the capacity to change and challenge attitudes and understandings of the perspective of the research subject and to make links between past lives and present experience as well as hopes for the future.

In what follows I will be looking at definitions of life history, at examples of research using this approach and then, with the help of two transcribed excerpts, I will look at some issues relating to the collection and analysis of life history data.

Definitions

The turn to biography in social science (Chamberlayne *et al.* 2000) coupled with a more open, sometimes grudging, acceptance of the contribution of memory in historical research (Thompson 2000: Chapter 2) has resulted in a proliferation of terms, schools and groupings often used interchangeably, some with a disciplinary base, others attempting to carve out new territory between disciplines. Labels such as oral history, biography, life story, life history, narrative analysis, reminiscence and life review jostle and compete for attention. What is common to all is a focus on the recording and interpretation, by some means or other, of the life experience of individuals. Though there are shared concerns, and, to an extent, shared literatures, there are differences in approach and in methods of data collection and analysis.

Oral history and life history

One way of grouping these different labels is in terms of their relation to the subject, the informant, interviewee or respondent. Oral history, life history, reminiscence and life review tend to focus on the idea of the interviewee as an active participant in the research process. The conscious and willing participation of the person being interviewed means that the nature and conduct of the interview itself becomes a dominant feature of the research process. In addition, a focus on outcomes which attempts to maintain engagement with participants has, historically, also been a key feature. Oral history with its background in democratic and emancipatory forms of historical research and history making involving women and working-class people in the late 1960s and 1970s has continued its radical stance in more recent times with histories of people with learning difficulties, migrants, mental health survivors, indigenous peoples and other marginalized groups (Thomson *et al.* 1994). Among its aims, as Michael Frisch explains (1990), are the exploration of 'more history', the revelation of aspects of the past not previously acknowledged or accessible through conventional documentary sources and 'anti-history', which he describes as an attempt to bypass academic scholarship by speaking directly to those with real authority, witnesses to the past.

Where oral history draws on memory and testimony to gain a more complete or different understanding of a past experienced both individually and collectively (Thompson 2000), life history takes the individual life and its told history with a view to understanding social processes determined by class, culture and gender, for example, drawing on other sources of data, survey-based, documentary, personal, public and private, to elaborate the analysis (Bertaux 1982). The difference between the two is very fine and the two terms are often used interchangeably.

A third and related approach sees the life story and its telling as the main focus, exploring patterns of narration and details of chronology, and identifying what is common or specific to other, similarly generated, accounts. By focusing on individual life stories researchers seek out similarities and differences which help to reveal decisions, opportunities, constraints and actions taken.

Evidence from life history work, which is what I am focusing on in this chapter, can be used to explore generational changes, shifts in language and expression, cohort experiences and relationships between individual agency and social structure. A life history approach may draw on a range of sources, including, as well as interviews, autobiographical writing, diaries, memoirs and a range of subjectively founded accounts. Both oral history and life history, as Ken Plummer argues, draw on 'researched and solicited stories . . . (which) do not naturalistically occur in everyday life; rather they have to be seduced, coaxed and interrogated out of subjects . . .' (Plummer 2001: 28). Both oral history and life history share common disciplinary heritages in history and sociology, though the influences of psychology and gerontology are increasingly playing a part (Thompson 2000; Bornat 2001).

Biographical and narrative analysis

In contrast, biographical and narrative approaches to life story telling tend to be characterized by analyses which place great emphasis on the deployment of psychoanalytically based theorizing during and after the interview at the stage of data analysis. As Robert Miller suggests, the narrative interview is understood in terms of the individual's conscious and subconscious 'composing and constructing a story the teller can be pleased with' (2000: 12). From this perspective the interview is understood as a social relationship in which 'Questions of fact take second place to understanding the individual's unique and changing perspective' (Miller 2000: 13). The contribution of the researcher to this process is spelled out by Wendy Hollway and Tony Jefferson:

> As researchers . . . we cannot be detached but must examine our subjective involvement because it will help us to shape the way in which we interpret interview data. This approach is consistent with the emphasis on reflexivity in the interview, but it understands the subjectivity of the interviewer through a model which includes unconscious, conflictual forces rather than simply conscious ones . . .
> (Hollway and Jefferson 2000: 33)

Such an approach, though it allows for active reconstruction and fluidity in the telling of a story, inevitably draws on the theoretical framework employed in its explanation. Paradoxically, given the focus on subjectivity and theorizing the perception of the individual, it may shift the balance of power away from the teller and towards the interpreter.

Silences and the subject

Drawing up distinctions and definitions can lead to false boundary construction. It would be wrong to present oral history and life history approaches to interviewing as ignorant of the social relations of the interview or of the varied subjectivities of the interviewee. Lusia Passerini has discussed how 'silences' in workers' accounts of the fascist 1920s in Italy left her baffled until she understood how these pointed to the reality of their daily experience and the need to adjust her own understanding of life at that time (Passerini 1998: 59–60). Al Thomson's research with Anzac survivors of the First World War took him into an exploration of the ways in which these very old men had lived with experiences which at times had contrasted with the public account and yet had arrived at a 'composure' which enabled them to tell their stories in ways that felt comfortable and recognizable to themselves and to Thomson, their interviewer (Thomson 1994: 9–12). In a collaborative interview with Linda Lord, a former poultry worker, Alicia Rouverol argues that what appears as a 'richly layered, seemingly contradictory narrative' provides a more complete understanding of what losing your job means (Rouverol 2000). Feminist oral historians and ethnographers helped to shift the focus towards the subject by initiating debates which explored the relationship between interviewer and interviewee, raising questions about shared identity, oppression and ownership as well as voice and perspective (see for example Personal Narratives Group 1989; Gluck and Patai 1991; Sangster 1998).

Reminiscence and life review

Reminiscence and life review are related approaches which at times are used interchangeably with oral history and life history. What distinguishes them is their development in relation to work with older people. Where reminiscence is the focus then the activity of remembering tends to be directed more towards the achievement of an outcome for the speaker or speakers involved. Reminiscence, while it is also a normal part of everyday inner life, when it is encouraged on a group or individual basis seeks to evoke the past with a view to bringing about a change in, for example, mood, social interaction or feelings of self-worth. Life review is more likely to be carried out on a one-to-one basis with a professional or practitioner who seeks to help someone to understand and reflect their life as a whole, accepting it in all its aspects, as it has been lived (Bornat 1994: 3–4). As Jeff and Christina Garland explain, 'Review helps people to learn to know themselves and others, and to be more fully human' (2001: 3). Life review is more of an intervention than a research method. However, it is certainly the case that the life history or oral history interview often has a strong life review aspect within it. Interviewees sometimes express themselves as welcoming the opportunity to reflect and describe new understandings about themselves, others and events they have experienced.

In their study of ageing and growing older, Paul Thompson *et al.* identified a therapeutic aspect to their research, observing that the older people they spoke to used the interviews as part of a search for meaning in their late lives (1990: 245). In a study of older people and family change, which I will be drawing on in the next section, among other things the perspectives of older people helped to shape the approach to interviewing, and as the interviews emerged from transcription it became clear that, for many of the respondents, the opportunity to tell their story was enabling them to achieve certain late life tasks relating to issues such as generativity and reflection on past experience (Bornat *et al.* 2000).

I have indicated that there is a range of possible approaches to interviewing, but how has gerontology benefited from oral history and life history research?

Implications for gerontology

Malcolm Johnson's early plea for a biographical approach (1976) helped to initiate what is now an orthodoxy: the rich yield of biographical approaches to understanding old age and the experience of later life (Dant and Gearing 1990; Fairhurst 1997: Phillipson 1998: 23–7). His appeal came at a time when older people themselves were beginning to draw on their own experience as a source of evidence in campaigns to raise their standards of living and care. Gladys Elder, a pioneer campaigner in the 1970s, in *The Alienated: Growing Old Today* (1977) drew liberally on her own and other older people's life histories to make her case. In another genre, the poem 'Kate' or 'Crabbit old woman', which emerged at about the same time, continues to sustain the idea of biographical narrative as a key to understanding late life (Bornat, n.d.). Despite these early affirmations there have been few researchers who have taken a life history approach. Jenny Hockey and Allison James's study of cultural representations of youth and ageing (1993) takes a life course rather than a life history focus with the attention they give to life stages; however, they draw conclusions from observation rather than life history accounts.

In contrast, Katherine Allen (1989) with her study of single women and Chris Phillipson *et al.*'s (2000) comparative review of three English communities over fifty years draw on interview data which is strongly biographical. Margot Jefferys's study of the founders of the geriatric specialty is based on over 70 interviews which narrate the lives of the respondents (Jefferys 2000) and she took a strongly biographical approach in her reflection on her own ageing (Jefferys 1997). Smaller studies of grandparenting and of grandmotherhood have also drawn on life history interviews (see for example Dunn 1991; Bamford 1994; Cannon 2000; Dench 2000). Within gerontology the adoption of life history research methods has not been overwhelming, though the contribution of life review and reminiscence in work with older people (see Coleman, Chapter 9 this volume) is well understood.

The subjects of oral history and life history research tend to be older people, however it took some time before oral historians began to realize that by interviewing older people they were engaging with experiences of ageing (Thompson *et al.* 1990: 5). Even then, interviews and projects which encompass whole lives and which acknowledge the influence of the perspective from late life have not been numerous. Some exceptions include Steve Hussey's study of the meaning of ageing in rural culture and Thompson *et al.*'s interviews with 55 older people, linked to an earlier set of interviews and providing a transgenerational understanding of changing experiences of old age (1990). Elsewhere I have argued the need for oral history to become more sensitive to the perspective of older people, and for reminiscence-based approaches to maintain an informed and heightened awareness of historical evidence as a context for promoting and understanding remembering in late life (Bornat 2001).

Non-gerontologists have contributed to the development of research practice in this area. For example, Dorothy Atkinson's work with older people with learning difficulties (1997) uses life history as a method to investigate past lives and to expose experiences of institutional living. Her approach sustains the emancipatory tradition of oral history and life history work being strongly participative and 'bottom-up' in its operation. Accounts of disability developed from interviews with disabled people take a lifelong perspective, demonstrating changing attitudes, policies and experience, and carry strong messages about the social construction of disability identities. In one example, the integration of other sources, documentary and photographic, adds context to the told stories (Humphries and Holland 1992).

Why more gerontologists have not drawn on life history data remains something of a puzzle. Cost may well be a deterrent. Funders who are looking for value for money research may baulk at the economics of costing interview, transcription and data analysis time in favour of speedier quantitative studies or the more immediately available results from focus groups and structured interviews. Lack of familiarity with, or even straight prejudice against, qualitative methods may be an additional factor. Life history research inevitably involves small sample sizes, and added to this is what may appear to be idiosyncratic or subjectively based interpretations of the data. However, biographical approaches generally are experiencing something of a revival and expansion, particularly in the area of social policy and welfare research (Chamberlayne *et al.* 2000). As Hollway and Jefferson argue, generalizations about social phenomena can become self-fulfilling prophecies unless they recognize subjective experience and the very different and 'irreducible character' of individual lives (2000: 127). Among postgraduate students the approach is certainly popular, and the support of a burgeoning literature formalizing and identifying replicable methods and procedures for life history data analysis suggests that the work of a new generation may well help to swell the number of sources available (see for example Clarke 2001).

In the next section I will explore issues for life history research with a case study from a funded project which drew extensively on life history interviews.

Case study

The 'stepfamily' project

In what follows I will outline how a life history approach was used in a project researching family change. Beginning with an outline of the rationale for the use of life histories I will then go on to look at the findings, drawing on the interview data to illustrate key points. Finally I look at some implications to be drawn from the experience.

The topic and the method

As part of a larger research programme[1] colleagues and I set out to investigate the implications for older people of the coterminosity of two sets of statistics: the ageing of the population and the rate of family change through divorce and separation. By the mid-1990s the proportion of the population over the age of 65 had reached 15 per cent, while in England and Wales four in every ten marriages were expected to end in divorce (Haskey 1996; OPCS 1996).

These statistics raised questions for us about the nature of intergenerational relationships, the care and support of more frail older family members and issues of inheritance and the sharing of family assets. In designing the research we chose a method, the unstructured life history interview, because we felt this would allow people to use their own language to describe the changes they were experiencing. We were keen to identify meanings attributed to family used over people's lifetimes and also to avoid any fixed notion of what might be happening by the use of terms such as 'stepfamily' (Bornat *et al.* 1999b: 252 ff).

Though we had identified a set of questions we had no prior theories which we were testing. This is very much an emergent area of study which, as we began, had only a small literature attached to it, hence the need for an inductive approach which would enable us to develop our understanding and further shape our own ideas as to what might be happening as the data were analysed. The perspectives of those directly involved in family change were important to us. They were actors, with agency and views on what they were experiencing (Miller 2000: 11). We were keen to enable people to reflect on their own lives over time and to be able to make comparisons, both generational and personal. For these reasons the life history interview presented itself as the ideal instrument.

Family change issues, with helpful examples provided by the royal family, were much debated in the media at the time, but their full implications were still emergent in many ways. For this reason in seeking respondents we deliberately chose a wording, 'family change', which, in its looseness, made no assumptions as to type of relationship and which we felt was non-judgemental. We were as much interested in *how people* told their stories as in *what* they told us (for a more detailed account of our sampling procedure see Bornat *et al.* 1999a).

Because we were interested in gaining the views of people from different generations our final total of 60 interviewees included people ranging in age from their early twenties to their late eighties. These comprised eight 'younger' people, that is people under 30 years of age with and without dependent children and with living parents and grandparents, 33 'middle-aged' people between 30 and 59 years of age with and without dependent children and dependent parents, and 31 'older' people over 60 years of age with children and grandchildren but no living parents.

The life history interviews were unstructured although the interviewers probed areas concerning the project topics: intergenerational relationships; caring arrangements and transfers of family resources. The interviews tended to be around an hour and half long, though some were shorter and longer than this. All were conducted in people's own homes, mainly alone, though a number of couples were interviewed together. As a funded project one of the team members was the paid researcher and carried out most of the interviews though each member of the team also carried out interviews at some stage.

After the interviews had been completed each interviewee was given a consent and clearance form to sign. This assigned copyright to the 'Stepfamily Project', a necessary stage if material is to be used in a publication.[2] We also informed respondents that we intended depositing the interview data with Qualidata[3] and asked them to specify their preferences as to access. The majority of those who responded (some interviewees were untraceable despite many attempts to contact them up to a year later) gave consent for their interviews to be deposited with Qualidata. Only four stipulated use by the project only and no archiving. What may feel like rather formal procedures, described here, are necessary, both legally and ethically. They help respondents to feel secure and comfortable with the research process and they also help researchers to document and keep track of their sample afterwards.

All the interviews were fully transcribed and analysed using a grounded theory approach (Glaser and Strauss 1967; Gilgun 1992) which identified underlying themes within the data as well as a focus which emphasized consideration of the language used in relation to family change. Grounded theory tends to be the method of choice for most people working with life history data. If the steps in data analysis are made transparent and are explained it provides the most secure means to guaranteeing a method which, while it deliberately makes use of researcher insight and reflection, guards against allegations of subjectivity and lack of generalizability or theoretical relevance (Wengraf 2001: 92–5).

Debates about grounded theory method focus, among other things, on the extent to which prior theories or even hypotheses are allowable given that analysis of the data is seen as a process of inductive theory generation. In the stepfamily case, as I have shown, we began with some questions about the outcomes of the association of divorce rates and an ageing population. In addition we had identified three issues which we thought would shed light on how families were responding to these changes. It was with this rather loose framework in mind that we embarked on the analysis of our data.

The data

Our interviews were professionally transcribed, presenting us with many hours of listening and pages of text for analysis. Though we chose our transcriber with care, seeking someone with sympathy for the subject as well as an ear for differing speech cadences and the dynamics of the interview, this did put some of the team at a disadvantage if they had not heard the original interview. A transcription is only a version of the recorded voices; the interviewer will always have a more complete sense of the emotions behind the words in the text (Yow 1994: 227 and ff). Ideally the whole team might have listened to all the tapes. This was not possible given our schedule and its time limits.

Our approach was to read and reread the whole transcript and to discuss emergent ideas and themes within the context of the whole life as narrated and described in the interview. Ideas and categories were compared and reviewed against the accounts we had collected as we searched for confirmations and contradictions of issues relating to family change by identifying common instances as well as uniquely telling accounts. The value of a life history approach lies in the opportunity it provides to take the whole life as well as wider socioeconomic and historical contexts into consideration when analysing the data. We might, for example, see how a particular experience of being a child was later followed up in becoming a parent while at the same time reading up for contextual reasons the social history of the Second World War or the decline of the straw hat trade in Luton (where we carried out our fieldwork) and exploring the literature on attachment in later life.

To accompany the transcripts a genogram of three to four generations was constructed drawing on the events and names mentioned by the interviewee. These helped us to make sense of what were often complicated family relationships and also contributed to our discussions and the generation of themes.

Working through the transcripts in discussions, a number of themes emerged in relation to our three areas of interest: intergenerational relations; the distribution of family assets; and care relationships. We began to find examples of how people talked about these issues as well as the evaluations which they were making, in particular how they had adapted to unexpected happenings and were managing family change privately and publicly.

Intergenerational relationships

Reading through the accounts we were struck by the ways in which people were continuing to preserve a parental role until late ages. This was evident both in terms of the ways in which people made moral statements about their children's actions and in what they told us about their reactions to events in their families. The gerontological literature stresses 'caring for' roles in families, with older people rather the passive subjects of caring decisions; however, our older interviewees, in commenting on the changes that they had seen or were experiencing, were clearly continuing to see themselves in parental roles. The conclusion we drew from this was that 'You're never too old to be a parent.'

For example, Wilma Walden,[4] an 86-year-old woman who had divorced during the Second World War and brought up three children until she married again, having five children in all from her two marriages and with a daughter and granddaughter also divorced, when asked how she hoped things would be for her family replied:

> Yes, you wish they could be the same as us, you know. See but I suppose some parents, they're not all the same, you know. The thing is, parents, they should never interfere with the children when they're married. Because they've got their lives to live, but you're there, when they want you, you're there, and they're there, when we want. Because they've all got their own little lives, haven't they? – when they're married. And that's how we like it. I mean, I'm on the phone, I can reach any of them and they'll be up here in a minute if I wanted them. Any of them . . .

And, contrasting her own family with others,

> They drift apart, don't they? They often drift apart, you see. But we're so close, and, you know, we've all helped each other, and like, and have been there when they wanted them, like, and – the thing is, all of them are stuck to me and C. [second husband]. See. That's how it's

been all the way through. I mean, I know I helped them. You know, if they want any help and if I've got a few bob and they're hard up – that's how it's been. I've always been able to help them.

Molly Lowe, living with her husband of fifty years and mother to eight children, among whom one daughter was divorced, another was widowed and a son was married to a divorced Catholic, discussed her feelings towards her ex-son-in-law:

See it wasn't right. I don't know. Perhaps he'd got a problem. But I'm afraid he had to sort it out. I could only look for our side. Although I don't always sympathize with our own children. They're our children, we know what makes them tick. And normally we're more for the in-laws, inasmuch as – not sympathize, but we can try and understand those. I always said, we know our own children, we know what makes them tick and what their problems are. But no, we tried with him, we really did. I mean he was welcomed into the family. He'd got no interest in the girls. And it was sad, very sad.

The moral tone adopted by Molly Lowe was also, we felt, a not untypical example of continuing to parent, remaining attached to the parenting role and to the children. Several of our interviewees made comments which showed that although they were not prepared to withdraw affection from their grown-up children they might not approve of their actions towards their partners and spouses. In her account Molly Lowe makes much of her own parents' divorce and reflects on her children's experience by recalling her own painful feelings at the time. Drawing on her life history was an active process for her during the interview and she used incidents from that period in her life to illustrate and support her way of accounting for her parenting style.

Noting such active parenting roles late in life helps to broaden out perceptions of the lives of older family members. Even those like Wilma Walden who were dependent on their children and grandchildren for support and social contact could still retain an identity as parents with opinions and experience to draw on. Often their experience provided them with more sympathy than might be expected given the rather rapid change which they had experienced in relation to marriages and partnerships within their own families and society generally.

The distribution of family assets and care relationships

Briefly, our analysis of the interviews using a life history approach enabled us to draw out new themes for the two other issues which interested us. In relation to the distribution of family assets, we asked our interviewees about how they wanted their assets to be divided after their death. Evidence from other studies (Finch and Wallis 1994) suggests that the urge to be viewed as a 'good parent' tends to mean that possessions will be divided equally among children, irrespective of need or strategic rewarding. In this way 'fairness' serves as a dominant morality, as children are stripped of their accumulated assets and treated almost as juvenile dependents once more.

Though some families were at quite different points in their reconstitution, and some had step-relationships over more than a generation whereas others were quite recently formed, it seemed that, in whatever case, parents sought to emphasize blood lines more prominently. The exercise of 'fairness' seemed to be a strong urge where parenting ties might have appeared to be undermined by the introduction of stepchildren into families. 'Fairness', 'shared' and 'equally' recurred with great frequency in the accounts of the interviews in this study.

Reading through the transcripts for references to care revealed many different themes including issues around reciprocity, obligation, choice and burden. The people we interviewed were well versed in many of the issues which gerontologists have concerned themselves with. However, we also found that taking a life history approach enabled us to identify ways in which caring relationships had an emotional history and could be determined by gendered expectations.

We detected what we saw as the emergence of the feminization of the family. The quality and durability of family ties appeared to be restricted in scope and dependent on the quality of relationships between women. Listening to the men talking about care and support reinforced this perception. Men talked much less about their involvement in intergenerational relationships even when they were adopting more 'modern' attitudes to careers and child care arrangements. It therefore seems likely that only those who have women partners were likely to be saved from exclusion in situations following family change.

While a life history approach was helpful to us in identifying context and rationales for experiences and decision making, and provided us with richly detailed data about the experience of family change over three generations, it did not provide us with conclusive evidence as to durability of the changes in attitudes and decisions which were reported to us. For example, was the feminist language of the younger women a cohort characteristic which they will retain, or is it a life stage characteristic which will ultimately be supplanted as they in turn grow older and a 'mature feminization' of the family takes over? Are they speaking in the language of the age they live in or the language of the age they are at?

The life history data suggests that what we were hearing was a combination of the two. With life experience of family change over more than one generation and a changing context for marriage and divorce generally, older people manage their hopes and expectations for support and independence with a mix of traditional and evolving emotions and reflections. Some of our oldest interviewees displayed a flexibility of attitude coupled with continuing involvement in the issues of partnering and family relationships.

The project which I have just described was carried out as a piece of academic research. Other projects with different funding constraints have followed up with outputs which reach wider sections of the community. For example, edited collections of interviews, both printed and recorded, life story books as well as local seminars and meetings have all been used to enable the voices of contributors to be heard across a range of media. This may not always be the choice of interviewees and a sensitive approach to dissemination will help to identify how people would prefer their voices to be heard. In the end, emancipation and empowerment should be developed in such a way that all feel satisfied and appropriately represented and served.

Implications

What lessons can be learned from this particular example of working with life history data? In particular, what are the advantages and disadvantages?

The advantages included:

- rich interview data yielding individual accounts of family change, historical data and examples of language and expression as well as opinion and analysis;
- linking individual life choices, opportunities and agency to broader structural divisions and change;
- opportunities to make sense of the demographics of family change at an individual level;
- opportunities to hear in people's own words how they work through issues of family change;
- manual analysis of the data keeps researchers closer to the original data;
- software packages help to save and manage time during data analysis.

Disadvantages which could be identified include:

- time taken in interviewing and transcription can slow the process of analysing and reviewing the development of ideas as the project developed;
- interviewees may not always appreciate the reasons for taking a life history approach to contextualize what they have identified as a specific problem or experience;
- the generation of a richly detailed data set presents challenges for management whether by one person or a team;

- familiarity with the contexts of life history experience – historical, socio-economic, cultural, demographic – requires allocating time for relevant literatures;
- manual analysis of the data can be time-consuming;
- the use of software packages can result in fragmentation and loss of control over narrative structures and in the generation of insights.

Practical suggestions

Effective life history research depends on awareness and development of certain skills. As in any research project, awareness of how to budget for different items will be helpful. For example, life history research means that you will be working with technical equipment and will need to budget for consumables such as tapes or minidisks as well as transcription time. Costs can mount up once you know that you should allow between five and seven hours to transcribe an hour of recorded time. This is one practical reason why people sometimes prefer to carry out their own transcribing, though this means extending the project in other ways by allocating sufficient time. Budgeting should include enough for copies to be made of each interview. One copy should be kept as a master, the other used for transcribing and editing. Interviewing skills in listening, question framing and empathizing are clearly essential.

Sensitivity in dealing with what may turn out to be 'difficult' areas and awareness of how to engage and disengage in ways which are supportive and non-threatening to participants are also a necessary part of the repertoire of interviewing skills (Yow 1994; Hollway and Jefferson 2000; Thompson 2000).

It is helpful to keep a well-organized administrative base for life history research. For example, details of all interviewees – their contact details, when first approached, when interviewed and last seen – should be included alongside records of their responses to requests for the release of their interviews, summaries of their interviews and copies of their transcripts, original and amended.

Projects involving life history work must include adequate time for data analysis. As a rough guide, approximately a quarter of any time schedule should be allocated for this phase, whether or not the process is handled manually or with the aid of a software package.

Whether you are working on your own or with a team, it is helpful to keep a close track or audit of the generation of your insights into the data. A research diary is essential as part of this process and should include reflections on what happens at each stage of the process.

A final point may be the deposit of any recordings which are made. Though this rounds off the project it is something which needs to be sorted out at an early stage. For example, details of possible archives should be identified, together with notes about what information is required as well as any protocols for anonymizing the recordings.

Conclusion

Within gerontology, life history research has so far not been well developed at the level of the survey. Most studies have drawn on fairly small samples or have been developed in relation to practice developments, linked to other research strategies.

Opportunities to draw across from life history into gerontology help to broaden out contexts for ageing across the life course, while drawing gerontology into life history helps to highlight the experience and tasks of ageing in interviews with older people.

Life history work brings with it a reputation for a more emancipatory and empowering approach to data collection about ageing. The resulting data tends to be rich in content and in opportunities for interpretation and different representational forms.

Any disadvantages tend to emerge in relation to costs and resourcing; short-term projects are not an ideal framework for this method. This combination of factors means that underinformed funders tend to question the relationship between costs and size of samples.

Used in conjunction with other methods, including documentary research and large data sets, it provides opportunities for links to be demonstrated between individual decision making and choice within broader structural and historical constraints. The results can be shown to have implications for social policy debates and practice development across a wide range of settings.

Notes

1 Bornat, Dimmock, Jones and Peace, 'The impact of family change on older people: the case of stepfamilies', ESRC reference number L31523003. The project was part of the 'Household and Family Change' programme.
2 When an interview is recorded, separate copyright in the words spoken and the recording are created (Copyright Act 1988). The owner of the copyright in the words is the speaker. Ownership in the recording belongs to the person or organization responsible for the making of the recording. This might be individuals working on their own, or it could be their employer or another organization. In order for the written transcript of interviews to be used, the owner – the person who spoke the words – should assign copyright to the person who seeks to make use of them. This only refers to the words spoken at that time, of course. Assigning copyright does not mean that those same words or accounts cannot be spoken again and owned in other transcriptions.

For details of copyright law and an example of a clearance and consent form see the Oral History Society website (Appendix), under 'Copyright and ethics'.

3 Qualidata is the ESRC Qualitative Data and Archive Resource Centre at the Department of Sociology, University of Essex. It was set up to facilitate and document the archiving of qualitative data arising from research. See Appendix for website address.

4 All names from the Stepfamily survey used here are pseudonyms.

References

Allen, K. (1989) *Single Women/Family Ties: The Life Histories of Older Women*. London: Sage Publications.

Atkinson, D. (1997) *An Auto/Biographical Approach to Learning Disability Research*. Aldershot: Ashgate.

Bamford, C. (1994) *Grandparents' Lives: Men and Women in Later Life*. Edinburgh: Age Concern Scotland.

Bertaux, J. (1982) The life course approach as a challenge to the social sciences, in T.K. Hareven and K.J. Adams (eds) *Ageing and Life Course Transitions: An Interdisciplinary Perspective*, pp. 127–50. London: Tavistock.

Bornat, J. (n.d.) Finding Kate. Unpublished paper.

Bornat, J. (ed.) (1994) *Reminiscence Reviewed: Perspectives, Evaluations, Achievements*. Buckingham: Open University Press.

Bornat, J. (2001) Reminiscence and oral history: parallel universes or shared endeavour? *Ageing and Society*, 21: 219–41.

Bornat, J., Dimmock, B., Jones, D. and Peace, S. (1999a) Stepfamilies and older people: evaluating the implications of family change for an ageing population, *Ageing and Society*, 19(2): 239–61.

Bornat, J., Dimmock, B., Jones, D. and Peace, S. (1999b) The impact of family change on older people: the case of stepfamilies, in S. McRae (ed.) *Changing Britain: Families and Households in the 1990s*, pp. 248–62. Oxford: Oxford University Press.

Bornat, J., Dimmock, B., Jones, D. and Peace, S. (2000) Researching the implications of family change for older people: the contribution of a life history approach, in P. Chamberlayne, J. Bornat and T. Wengraf (eds) *The Turn to Biographical Methods in Social Science: Comparative Issues and Examples*, pp. 244–60. London: Routledge.

Cannon, C. (ed.) (2000) *Our Grandmothers, Our Mothers, Ourselves*. London: Third Age Press.

Chamberlayne, P., Bornat, J. and Wengraf, T. (2000) *The Turn to Biographical Methods in Social Science*. London: Routledge.

Clarke, A. (2001) Looking back and looking forward: a biographical approach to ageing. Unpublished PhD, University of Sheffield.

Dant, T. and Gearing, B. (1990) Doing biographical research, in S. Peace (ed.) *Researching Social Gerontology*, pp. 143–59. London: Sage Publications/BSG.

Dench, G. (2000) *Grandmothers of the Revolution*. London: Hera Trust with Institute for Community Studies.

Dunn, N. (1991) *Grandmothers*. London: Chatto and Windus.

Elder, G. (1977) *The Alienated: Growing Old Today*. London: Writers and Readers Publishing Co-operative.

Fairhurst, E. (1997) Recalling life: analytical issues in the use of 'memories', in A. Jamieson, S. Harper and C. Victor (eds) *Critical Approaches to Ageing and Later Life*, pp. 62–73. Buckingham: Open University Press.

Finch, J. and Wallis, L. (1994) Inheritance care bargains and elderly people's relationships with their children, in D. Challis, B. Davies and K. Traske (eds) *Community Care: New Agendas and Challenges*, pp. 110–19. Aldershot: Ashgate/British Society of Gerontology.

Frisch, M. (1990) *A Shared Authority: Essays on the Craft and Meaning of Oral and Public History*. New York, NY: SUNY.

Garland, J. and Garland, C. (2001) *Life Review in Health and Social Care: A Practitioner's Guide*. Hove: Brunner-Routledge.

Gilgun, J.F. (1992) Definitions, methodologies, and methods in qualitative family research, in J.F. Gilgun, D. Daly and G. Handel (eds) *Qualitative Methods in Family Research*, pp. 22–39. London: Sage Publications.

Glaser, B.G. and Strauss, A.L. (1967) *The Discovery of Grounded Theory: Strategies for Qualitative Research*. New York, NY: Aldine de Gruyter.

Gluck, S.B and Patai, D. (eds) (1991) *Women's Words: The Feminist Practice of Oral History*. London: Routledge.

Haskey, J. (1996) The proportion of married couples who divorce: past patterns and current prospects, *Population Trends*, 83: 25–36.

Hockey, J. and James, A. (1993) *Growing Up and Growing Old*. London: Sage Publications.

Hollway, W. and Jefferson, T. (2000) *Doing Qualitative Research Differently*. London: Sage Publications.

Humphries, S. and Holland, P. (1992) *Out of Sight: The Experience of Disability 1900–1950*. Plymouth: Northcote House.

Jefferys, M. (1997) Inter-generational relationships: an autobiographical perspective, in A. Jamieson, S. Harper and C. Victor (eds) *Critical Approaches to Ageing and Later Life*, pp. 77–89. Buckingham: Open University Press.

Jefferys, M. (2000) Recollections of the pioneers of the geriatric medicine specialty, in J. Bornat, R. Perks, P. Thompson and J. Walmsley (eds) *Oral History, Health and Welfare*, pp. 5–97. London: Routledge.

Johnson, M. (1976) 'That was your life': a biographical approach to later life, in J.M.A. Munnichs and W.V.A. van den Heuval (eds) *Dependency and Interdependency in Old Age*, pp. 147–61. The Hague: Nijhoff.

Miller, R.L. (2000) *Researching Life Stories and Family Histories*. London: Sage Publications.

OPCS (Office of Population Censuses and Surveys) (1996) *Living in Britain: Results from the 1994 General Household Survey*. London: HMSO.

Passerini, L. (1998) Work ideology and consensus under Italian fascism, in R. Perks and A. Thomson (eds) *The Oral History Reader*, pp. 53–62. London: Routledge.

Personal Narratives Group (1989) (eds) *Interpreting Women's Lives: Feminist Theory and Personal Narratives*. Indiana, IN: Indiana University Press.

Phillipson, C. (1998) *Reconstructing Old Age: New Agendas in Social Theory and Practice*. London: Sage Publications.

Phillipson, C., Bernard, M., Phillips, J. and Ogg, J. (2000) *The Family and Community Life of Older People: Social Networks and Social Support in Three Urban Areas*. London: Routledge.

Plummer, K. (2001) *Documents of Life*. London: Sage Publications.

Rouverol, A. (2000) 'I was content and not content', *Oral History*, 28(2): 66–78.

Sangster, J. (1998) Telling our stories: feminist debates and oral history, in R. Perks and A. Thomson, *The Oral History Reader*, pp. 87–100. London: Routledge.

Thompson, P. (2000) *The Voice of the Past*, 3rd edn. Oxford: Oxford University Press.

Thompson, P., Itzin, C. and Abendstern, M. (1990) *I Don't Feel Old: The Experience of Later Life*. Oxford, Oxford University Press.

Thomson, A. (1994) *Anzac Memories: Living with the Legend*. Oxford: Oxford University Press.

Thomson, A., Frisch, M. and Hamilton, P. (1994) The memory and history debates: some international perspectives, *Oral History*, 22(2): 33–43.

Wengraf, T. (2001) *Qualitative Research Interviewing*. London: Sage Publications.

Yow, V.R. (1994) *Recording Oral History: A Practical Guide for Social Scientists*. London: Sage Publications.

9

Doing case study research in psychology

Peter Coleman

Introduction

The case study has been called 'the bedrock of scientific investigation' (Bromley 1986: ix). Yet it has been surprisingly little used in psychological research. McAdams points out the irony 'that the field defined as the scientific study of the individual person should harbour deep ambivalence about the very business of examining cases of individual persons' lives' (McAdams and West 1997: 761).

There was an active tradition of case study in personality carried out in the USA between the wars by such distinguished psychologists as Henry Murray and Gordon Allport (Allport 1937; Murray 1938), but its value was overlooked in the postwar enthusiasm for quantitative methods. The recovery of case study research within psychology in recent years has been more restrained than in other social sciences (see for example Yin 1984; Hartley 1994; Stake 1994; Keen and Packwood 1995). Still relatively few case study investigations are reported in the major psychological journals (the *Journal of Personality* is one of the few which does publish lengthy case analyses). For this reason the use of case study in psychological research has to be carefully explained and justified to an audience which is still generally sceptical as to its value. This applies particularly to PhD and other graduate studies where the pressures for conservatism in methodology are most marked. But fortunately there has been sufficient discussion of case study method in the recent psychological literature to provide the necessary respectability and, more importantly, reflective awareness to case-based graduate research in psychology (e.g. Alexander 1990; Bromley 1990, 1991; Runyan 1990, 1997; Edwards 1998).

The low status of case study investigations is reflected in the lesser scientific status given to clinical and other applied studies in psychology where case studies have always played a role (Shapiro 1966). But there are now distinct signs of a recovery of confidence on the part of case study researchers working especially in applied areas. Daniel Fishman's (1999) *The Case for Pragmatic Psychology* is a confident assault on the hegemony of the quantitative approach to explaining human behaviour. He argues that the cumulative study of individual cases will provide better practical answers to most psychological questions than the abstract analysis of a matrix of variables. Researchers in clinical psychology, educational, social and other applied fields, including gerontology, should no longer need feel second-class citizens if they build up their enquiries on the basis of the study of individual lives. Rather they can regard themselves as providing a model for future psychological research that gives due recognition to context and meaning in human lives.

Definitions and key issues in case study analysis

In the middle of the last century, when the practice of individual personality investigation was common in psychology, the debate between case study and quantitative variable analysis was referred to in terms of 'idiographic' versus 'nomothetic' research (i.e. describing the individual case and postulating a rule or generalization). The most common criticism made of psychobiography and other forms of idiographic analysis was over the issue of generalization, that general rules could not be formulated on the basis of studying particular cases in isolation. In the 1950s and 1960s personality psychologists displayed growing optimism about the potential of quantitative analysis of large data sets. Thus Levy was able to describe as the primary goal of psychology 'the development of generalizations of ever increasing scope, so that greater and greater varieties of phenomena may be explained by them, larger and larger numbers of questions answered by them, and broader and broader reaching predictions and decisions based upon them' (Levy 1970: 5).

In reply the personologists argued for different levels of analysis within psychology (Runyan 1984). It is possible to discover universal generalizations that cover all people. It is also possible to determine generalizations that can be made about types of people, characteristic reactions that apply to some but not to others. But there are also generalizations, laws and structures to the way that particular individuals behave. As Henry Murray expressed it, 'every person is in certain respects like all other persons, like some other persons, and like no other persons'. What is mistaken is to assume that each level can necessarily be reduced to the next and ultimately to the most general level. It is this kind of casual assumption of reductionism that leads people to argue that finding out about individuals is not interesting or worthy enough an activity to be called a science.

This is still the first and most important point to be made in justifying psychological study of the individual case. It is a very simple one. It is not about denying the criticism that the study of one individual case explains in itself little about people as a whole, but asserting that psychology is also about trying to understand the individual person. If we are really interested in making progress in understanding people as individuals, rather than as exemplifications of a series of generalizations abstractly expressed and not coherently related to one another, we need a different research approach to the standard nomothetic one.

Although this chapter is mainly concerned with qualitative analysis of case study material, it is important to remember that there is also a tradition of experimental analysis of the individual case in psychology which uses statistical analysis on multiple recordings of an individual's behaviour, typically to investigate the effects of an intervention (for example in the care of a person suffering from a mental disorder or disability) (e.g. Barlow and Hersen 1984). The first illustrative example of case analysis presented later also employs quantitative methods, namely content analysis of verbal categories occurring in letters and other written documents.

Also very important is the distinction between a case study and a psychobiography. A psychological case study examines an individual's behaviour over a limited time span; a psychobiography examines a whole life, or at least a substantial part of it. Analysis of people in the public eye is a popular and remunerative task nowadays. A psychobiography differs from a biography in that it involves 'the systematic use of psychological (especially personality) theory to transform a life into a coherent and illuminating story' (McAdams 1988: 2). Its successful execution requires considerable investment in obtaining information about a person's life and a disciplined approach to theory and analysis. Unfortunately, because of the large-scale abdication of psychology from case study work, the study of individuals has been mostly conducted by non-psychologists, and their work generally lacks psychological rigour. However, some do provide insightful applications of psychological theory.

Runyan (1984) provides a scholarly survey of psychobiographies and other psychological case analyses conducted up to the time of his review. He also explains the characteristics of case study enquiry which distinguish it from typical nomothetic investigations. Explanation at the individual level often occurs not through the deductive application of universal generalizations, but rather through processes as searching for individuals' reasons for acting in a particular way, through collecting as much information as possible about the individual and looking for patterns within it, and through organizing information about the case into an intelligible narrative. Most psychobiographies have been written about famous (or notorious) individuals, but could and should be composed about any person, given sufficient data. Robert White's 'Lives in Progress' is an example from the Murray-Allport tradition of case study research of such investment (White 1952, 1966, 1975), but unfortunately it is almost unique.

Common faults which have tended to give psychobiography a bad reputation include relying overmuch on inadequate evidence, neglecting social and historical evidence, placing too much emphasis on childhood determinants, and overpathologizing behaviour. One of the examples of successful psychobiography that Runyan cites is Walter Jackson Bate's (1977) *Samuel Johnson*. There have been a number of psychobiographical analyses carried out on Dr Johnson, and this is largely thanks to the extensive and detailed contemporary source material provided by James Boswell's *The Life of Samuel Johnson* (Boswell [1791] 1968). This was written shortly after Johnson's death and drew on detailed written recordings that the author had made of his encounters with him. Boswell's biography remains a remarkable pioneering achievement because of the deliberate manner of its composition, its attempt to present Johnson whole and uncensored, and its search for additional reliable evidence from others who knew him (Sisman 2000). In this it is good biography, but this does not make it psychobiography, because there is no attempt at underlying theoretical explanation or interpretation for the development of Johnson's character. However, this is very much preferable to psychological theorizing on the basis of inadequate data.

Successful psychobiography requires many qualities, not only knowledge of history and of psychology, but also the subject's professional field, and some measure of literary skill. Runyan praises Bate's book 'for its expertise in historical enquiry, familiarity with Johnson's literary world and work, grasp of psychological theory, and grace in exposition' (Runyan 1984: 232). For example, Bate analyses well the origins of that high sense of self-demand and personal responsibility that Johnson displayed. Born the first child of older, protective parents, and suffering already in the first year of life from a tubercular infection of the lymph glands (scrofula) which left him with visual and hearing impairment, Johnson had to fight hard to develop autonomy of action. But Bate is careful not to overemphasize the pathological, but to bring out strengths and adaptive capacities as well, and formative influences not only in childhood but throughout the lifespan.

Runyan also cites favourably John E. Mack's (1976) study of 'Lawrence of Arabia' for its analysis of major themes in Lawrence's life and convincing narrative on how Lawrence coped with the problems which circumstances and his own characteristics led him into. Throughout all his adult life Lawrence was dogged by unresolved issues of identity which seemed to have stemmed from uncertainty about his parenthood. Yet these very difficulties gave him the capacity for empathy with all types of disadvantaged people. Mack was himself able to interview various people who spoke of Lawrence's ability to give them a sense of identity. In both these books one can see confirmation of the value of concepts in Erikson's lifespan developmental theory. Erikson himself wrote two notable psychobiographies on Luther and on Gandhi (Erikson 1958, 1969), both of which illustrate well his own theory of identity development (Erikson 1963).

In this chapter I shall continue to use illustrations from Erikson's theory, because of my own interest in its concepts and because I believe it to have particular and continued relevance for ageing. However, it is important not to confuse psychobiography with any particular theoretical viewpoint. There is a tendency to associate it with psychoanalysis because of the emphasis on psychodynamic theory found in many psychobiographies, starting with Freud's analysis of Leonardo da Vinci (Elms 1988). But in principle psycho-biographies, and case analyses, can be written from any theoretical viewpoint, even from behaviourist learning theory. Andrew Steptoe, Karen Reivich and Martin Seligman (1993), for example, provide an interesting short account of how they employed cognitive attribution analysis – examining the causal explanations people provide for events in their lives – to invest-igate Mozart's personality in his later years. Content analysis of his letters demonstrated that he continued to show high optimism and exuberant self-confidence in the face of difficulties.

A particularly intriguing approach to the study of whole lives is to exam-ine the accounts individuals have provided themselves of how the ends that they have sought during their lives have been transformed through experience, insight and the exercise of will (Freeman and Robinson 1990). A good example of this is the real-life case of Oskar Schindler, the hero of the film 'Schindler's List', whose original idea of employing Jewish labour in his factories for economic reasons during the Second World War became transformed into a plan to ensure their survival. In subsequent work Free-man has provided illuminating analyses of the processes involved in recon-sideration of identity at different stages of an individual's life and how a person comes to 'rewrite the self' in creating an autobiography (Freeman 1993). He has also examined the problems stemming from false identity, a realization that life has been lived without authentic meaning (Freeman 1997).

Although they appear as very different types of activities, there is an interdependence between nomothetic and idiographic levels of analysis. There can be both 'trickle-down' and 'ripple-up' effects. Psychobiography proceeds at least in part through the use of general theories in explaining individual lives. In fact analysis of the individual case constitutes an ideal testing ground for the value of new and old theories, as will be argued later. They provide a pragmatic test of whether one can actually use a theory in understanding an individual person's behaviour. Sometimes, very rarely, a general theory provides the missing piece in an otherwise incom-plete puzzle. Usually these are biological rather than psychological theories. Runyan uses the example of studies of King George III whose disturbed behaviour puzzled historians and other investigators for years until the discovery of the metabolic defect porphyria made it possible to explain much of his behaviour in these terms. The case of King George continues to interest case study researchers in psychology (Runyan 1988; Simonton 1998).

Examples of the ripple-up effects from the individual case to theorizing at the general level are provided by the lifespan theories on personality development of Jung on midlife change and of Erikson on identity crisis. Both reflect interpretations of their own life experience. But it is often not realized how, even in experimental and cognitive psychology, observation of the individual case provides the key to successful speculation on theory about human functioning. The type of exploratory case study analysis which can form the basis for new theory development is not illustrated in detail in this chapter, but its use is growing (Edwards 1998; Fishman 1999). It is obviously particularly applicable to new or little studied phenomena. Both validatory and exploratory case studies use similar principles of evidence and argument.

Execution and presentation of case studies

Despite the interdependence between ideographic and nomothetic research, the different levels of analysis and methods they use makes qualitative case study research and the examination of the interrelationship between variables within a population quite distinct types of research activity. The preoccupations are dissimilar. Issues of sampling, power calculation and significance testing dominate quantitative studies, whereas a central issue in both qualitative case study analysis and psychobiography is how one evaluates different and competing explanations of individuals' actions and the direction their lives take. To illustrate this point Runyan (1981) examined the many competing explanations that have been provided for why Vincent Van Gogh cut off his own ear and gave it to a prostitute. He indicates that it is possible to make progress with providing an explanation for this puzzling action even if it is not fully satisfactory. As in all scientific endeavours, explanations are progressive not absolute.

In the first place clear standards need to be set up for comparing different competing psychological interpretations. Such standards could be their logical soundness; their comprehensiveness in accounting for a number of puzzling aspects of the events in question; their survival of tests of attempted falsification, such as tests of derived predictions or retrodictions; their consistency with the full range of available relevant evidence; their support from above; or their consistency with more general knowledge about human functioning or about the person in question: their credibility relative to other explanatory hypotheses.

Thus Runyan shows how certain explanations (e.g. the influence on Vincent of newspaper reports concerning Jack the Ripper) have no evidence to support them, whereas others do (e.g. fascination with the action of the matador in giving the ear of the bull to the lady of his choice, and interest in depicting the scene in the Garden of Gethsemane where Simon Peter cuts off the ear of the servant of the chief priest). However, he gives the primary role in the explanation of Van Gogh's self-destructive action to his brother Theo's announcement of his impending marriage. He draws on evidence of Vincent's previous masochistic responses to rejection (e.g. by a young woman he had visited in the Netherlands) and subsequent mental breakdowns occasioned by Theo's actual marriage and the birth of his first child. He argues that at one important level of explanation it is possible to argue that Vincent cut off his ear in response to the perceived loss of, and rejection by, his brother.

In regard to Vincent Van Gogh's behaviour, as with many other well-recorded behaviours, i.e. where there is a lot of circumstantial evidence, one can make a reasonable attempt to come up with a theory. Satisfactory explanations may be found at one level of the analysis but not at another (e.g. why Van Gogh deliberately hurt himself; why he cut off his ear . . .). Some explanations will be more plausible than others. Often the reluctance to investigate the single case is due to the mass of evidence that has to be considered, not to any inherent improbability of reaching a conclusion. The collection of additional evidence on the case, and the development of new theories in psychology, may contribute further to understanding the behaviour.

Further discussion of the use of evaluative criteria in action can be found in the work of Dennis Bromley (1977, 1986, 1990, 1991), who compares the sifting of evidence for theories with that of the judicial process. The requirement on the investigator is to be both prosecutor and defence, to look for supporting and contrary evidence for different viewpoints. Finding corroboratory evidence is a particularly important consideration, just as in quantitative research there is a requirement of honesty and open-mindedness to obtaining results contrary to expectation.

An important point to bear in mind in writing case study analyses is that explanations of behaviour are not necessarily exclusive. So there is room for more than one good explanation for any given biographical event. Many events in life are highly overdetermined, and it is possible to trace how influences from many different levels may come to bear in producing a particular behaviour in a particular situation. The factors that have been identified are not all necessarily essential to bringing about the resulting action.

Human adjustment over a period of some months to a few years have been typical subjects of psychological case studies, and this makes the method of particular relevance to ageing. Bromley's 'quasi-judicial' method offers a suitably disciplined approach to the enquiry: establishing at the outset the precise nature of the question for investigation, assembling all the relevant evidence, deriving the most plausible conclusion from an unbiased consideration of all the evidence, and finally presenting that conclusion as coherently as possible together with the supportive evidence as well as with all the remaining caveats as to its validity.

Autobiographical material, as letters and diary accounts, provides a main source of data for psychobiographical and case study analysis, as will be illustrated later. A major problem often arises in reducing such data to manageable proportions. Obviously this has to be done systematically and in an unbiased way. This can be done by means of sampling as in nomothetic research, and examples of this method will be provided in a subsequent section. But sampling may lead to the neglect of unique but crucial data. A second method of data reduction is to select carefully material relevant to the specific orientation of one's study, for example relating to the person's present state of (mal)adjustment, as in the Van Gogh example cited above.

However, in more exploratory research of a psychobiographical character yet another approach is necessary to sifting data. Alexander (1988, 1990) suggests nine criteria or rules which can be employed to help to make a preliminary reduction of a large data set: primacy, frequency, uniqueness, negation, emphasis, omission, error or distortion, isolation, incompletion. Questioning the data in these ways (what comes first? what stands out? what seems to be missing? what does not follow logically?), and making the answers explicit, alerts the investigator to repetitive patterns of 'means–ends sequences', for example a person's responses to authority figures at different times of their life. Elucidating these behavioural sequences leads to the discovery of underlying themes – guiding motives and purposes – in the person's life narrative.

Use of case studies in testing and developing theory in lifespan development and ageing

Both examples of research which I wish to present to illustrate the psychological case study are concerned with the developmental study of adulthood and ageing. In addition both draw on the theoretical concepts of Erik Erikson. The first, more akin to a psychobiographical analysis, comprises a series of investigations into the documents (letters, diaries, novels) written by Vera Brittain, the British feminist and peace activist. They have been analysed by Abigail Stewart, Bill Peterson, Carol Franz and others, using Erikson's lifespan theory of sequential developmental tasks during adulthood. The second study, carried out by myself and colleagues, examines adjustment to ageing, in particular management of self-esteem and identity, in a number of individual cases selected from a larger longitudinal study of ageing. It thus provides an example of multi-case analysis. Both studies examine existing theory. The first investigates a theoretically related set of concepts which, although much referred to, have been relatively little investigated. The second study also draws on two strands of contrasting theorizing about the self in later life, one of which relates to identity, and compares their utility in illuminating cases especially selected for this purpose.

The potential of case studies for validating and developing theory needs clarification. In the ideographic tradition advocated by Allport and Murray, case-specific theories are formulated on the basis of systematic collection of evidence on a particular person, and tested by observation of subsequent behaviour. Such case analyses identify unique as well as common traits that characterize the person (Allport 1965). Lessons can be drawn from this case analysis and applied to the analysis of another person. Thus a theory, or more likely 'case-law', might be drawn up inductively around the analysis of the behaviour of a group of individuals. The 'case-law' typically would apply to a restricted range of situations, for example to people coping with a particular life adjustment such as a bereavement. But the primary focus of each analysis would be on understanding the persons themselves, and in terms which do justice to their individual character-istics. Subsequent generalization to a group or category of cases would be a secondary aim. As stated at the outset of this chapter, the primary justifica-tion of case study analysis is understanding of the individual.

However, it is also possible to examine how well a theory, for example in the area of personality functioning, applies to an individual case or to a group of cases. The theory, in these circumstances, would not be drawn inductively from the cases but from prior work, for example from clinical experience, from commonly accepted conceptualizations, or from the find-ings of nomothetic research. The strengths and weaknesses of the theory are highlighted in the attempt to apply them to the individual case. The first study examines one individual in this way. If a number of individuals are selected so as to represent a range of cases within the theory's domain, the critique that they together offer becomes the more compelling. The second study provides an example of such multi-case analysis. It is import-ant to be clear that in both the following studies the primary aim is to examine existing theory rather than develop new theory. However, it is of course possible that in testing existing theory such studies develop new theoretical notions as well. This is one advantage of the case study approach. Searching for understanding about individual persons by collect-ing evidence about them encourages the development of insight in a way that is impossible with statistical analysis.

Case studies

Case study 1: *Studies of Vera Brittain: the changing self*

Erikson's notion of identity connects individual and society:

> A sense of identity means a sense of being at one with oneself as one
> grows and develops; and it means, at the same time, a sense of affinity

with a community's sense of being at one with its future as well as its
history – or mythology.

(Head 1994: 325)

Identity, in Erikson's sense, also involves an existential sense of personal
well-being, that there is some purpose to one's life. Critics of Erikson's
concept point to the changed circumstances of modern societies in which
culture, community and belonging are less secure reference points. An
individual nowadays therefore has to negotiate a continuing sense of personal identity through changing currents. Erikson himself was well aware
of the changing nature of society and encouraged continued elaboration of
his ideas to relate better individual to social development.

Abigail Stewart's analysis (Stewart *et al.* 1988; Peterson and Stewart 1990)
of the writings of Vera Brittain, housed in the McMaster University Library,
Hamilton, Ontario, is consistent with this aim of theory development by
focused consideration on one person. Academic life rarely provides the
opportunity for adult lives to be studied over a long period of time. However, personal documents allow for a measure of concentrated retrospective analysis. Stewart set herself the task of seeing whether self-expressions
in Vera Brittain's writings developed over time in the way that Erikson's
theory would lead one to expect. In particular she wanted to analyse
the relative presence of themes of identity, intimacy and generativity, and
whether they followed the sequential order laid down in Erikson's
psychosocial stages, each stage building on the resolution of earlier stages.
The developmental path to psychosocial maturity suggested by Erikson
is from identity (the capacity to commit oneself to one's self) to intimacy
(the capacity to commit oneself to another individual) to generativity (the
capacity to commit to future generations).

Questions have been raised about the applicability of Erikson's theory
to women's development. Vera Brittain offered a particularly interesting
challenge, because of the feminist stance that she developed early in life.
She had fought her family's opposition to be allowed to follow her brother
to Oxford University and began studying English there in 1914. Her early
enthusiasm and sense of purpose was destroyed by the advent of the First
World War. At the end of her first year she left to contribute to the war
effort by nursing. Within a few months she had lost her fiancé, Roland, to
the war, and by the time the war ended she had lost her brother and other
good friends as well. She returned to Oxford where she changed her study
to history because it seemed more meaningful. She also became active in
internationalist and feminist groups. But she continued to suffer from a
continuing sense of futility and loss until eventually she found a vocation
in writing and lecturing. In this process she appears to have been helped by
meeting key friends including the man who was to become her husband.
For most of the remaining years of her life she continued to rework incidents and events from the war in her writings.

Throughout the war Brittain recorded her thoughts and feelings in a daily diary as well as in an extensive correspondence. To analyse it using Erikson's categories, Stewart and colleagues found they had to develop their own coding system. To do this they used an exhaustive review of Erikson's writings about each of the three stages, and from the statements they assembled they developed definitions for each major stage and reached a consensus on specific issues associated with each one. This process of definition is not a necessary requirement of case study research, since the concepts to be investigated may already be well operationalized. However, there are distinct advantages to working with concepts which one has fully digested oneself.

Using these definitions the raters found they were able to code with a very high level of category agreement. Sub-themes for identity included statements of sameness and continuity; identifications; occupational role; values; confirmation by friends and society; idealizations; awareness of characteristics and preferences. Intimacy themes included the willingness to fuse one's identity with that of another; the capacity to be faithful and committed to another person, recognizing their needs; a sense of connectedness, closeness and togetherness; and the concern for a mutually satisfying sexual relationship. Generativity themes included a preoccupation with caring for others; productivity; an inner awareness of one's need to be needed; and a concern about future generations.

They then proceeded to apply these codings to representative samples of text, using the meaningful phrase as the coding unit. Before coding they removed all references to date to avoid unconscious bias. In their first reported analysis (Stewart *et al.* 1988) they analysed Vera Brittain's experience from 1914 to 1916. Because the material was so extensive and because of the assumption that psychological change in adults occurs relatively slowly they decided to sample every fourth month. But in order to check this assumption all letters were coded covering a 7-month period including the crucial month of December 1915 in which she anticipated her fiancé's leave and learned of his death.

The major finding from this analysis is the overall pattern of intense concern with identity and far lesser concern with intimacy and generativity. This is consistent with Erikson's theory (but not with Brittain's autobiographical account written later in life, adopted also by some of her biographers, that during this period she experienced the central love of her life). Her preoccupations at the time were very much with her own opinions, values and future roles. However, it is also clear from the analysis that Roland's death precipitated a new identity crisis for her. The high point in identity concerns before Roland's death occurred shortly before her entrance to Oxford. Thereafter they declined until a steep rise immediately following his death.

Throughout the period of her relationship with Roland and after his death she expressed far less preoccupation with intimacy issues. This suggests to the researchers that it 'was not a fully mature, intimate relationship founded on two secure adult identities, but an adolescent relationship partially serving purposes of identity formation, at least for Brittain' (Stewart *et al.* 1988: 65). The patterns of scores for generativity suggest a slight trend toward increasing concern over the period, particularly linked to periods of positive commitment to nursing. In general the analysis supports Erikson's view that as a young adult Vera Brittain should have been consolidating an identity before facing issues of intimacy and generativity.

Subsequent analysis by Carol Franz (1995) showed that Vera Brittain's preoccupations with identity had declined by the age of 30 whereas concerns with intimacy and generativity rose. However, identity issues (especially relating to occupation) remained prominent. Peterson and Stewart (1990) report on her midlife concerns, making use not only of her diaries but also her novels. The latter is a more controversial use of personal material, but the logic behind it is the same as for other projective material like the Thematic Apperception Test (TAT) where people are asked to tell imaginative stories about ambiguous pictures (Morgan and Murray 1935), i.e. that we tend to express in fantasy the motives and issues that are important in our lives. The actual coded documents included Brittain's diary from 1932 to 1937 and from 1939 to 1944 and her five major fictional works, completed in 1922, 1924, 1936, 1944 and 1947. The scorer was blind to the dates of the material, the other researcher having randomly selected self-contained passages from the texts.

Many of the findings of this analysis are consistent with Erikson's theory, showing that Vera Brittain's overall identity and intimacy concerns declined significantly over time, while her overall generative concerns increased. During mature adulthood expressions of generativity appeared more often than expressions of intimacy, reversing the trend of young adulthood. However, in all the periods investigated identity concerns remained the predominant ones. Why, ask the authors, was Brittain still preoccupied with identity issues during mature adulthood? The personal documents of other individuals that have been analysed do not show this degree of permanent absorption with identity. However, examination of the diaries and letters of additional British writers of this period (Virginia Woolf, Siegfried Sassoon, Vita Sackville-West and Harold Nicolson) showed also a predominance of identity themes into midlife. Could this be a characteristic of writers?

Peterson and Stewart (1990) raise the possibility that this cohort, growing up in the social turmoil of the Great War and its aftermath, remained permanently preoccupied with identity. This is consistent with Erikson's interest in the influence of historical circumstances on individual development. Previous work by Stewart and Healy (1989) on women's participation in the labour force in the USA during the Second World War supports the view that the development of personality is shaped in part by social conditions. However, the psychological displacement caused by the First

World War was even greater than that of the Second World War. The former social stability had been destroyed and could not be rebuilt. The nationalistic and idealistic attitudes that people had formed in youth and which might be expected to last a lifetime were also overthrown, leading perhaps to a permanent search for worthy alternatives.

Vera Brittain proved to be a good choice for such studies of archival material. Of course the appropriateness of the type of archival material for investigating a particular subject has to be questioned. Perhaps diaries are less useful for investigating issues of intimacy and generativity than identity. To rely only on one source of data may be biasing. That is why there was a distinct advantage in both these studies of Vera Brittain's writings to include multiple sources: letters as well as diaries in the first, and novels in the second. The inclusion of the latter also proved worthwhile. Strong parallels were found between the expression of psychosocial themes in Brittain's diaries and novels written at the same time.

The practicalities of such analysis of documentation needs careful consideration. The task needs to be feasible in the time dimensions allowable. Therefore judicious selection may have to be applied. However, it is important to realize that this does not diminish the value of the exercise. Even if only a fraction of the material available can be considered, important psychosocial questions can be raised and perhaps answered.

Many opportunities for this type of research exist, particularly for the present older generation where documentary evidence often exists in the form of letters and diaries which can be utilized in studies of development and adjustment. Erikson's concepts are a good example of concepts which can be studied through writing, but there are many other theories in the developmental psychology of ageing which could be examined through case study analysis of existing written material. So far the method has usually been applied to the famous and deceased who are unwilling to (or cannot!) answer questions of clarification. Perhaps it is more challenging to investigate ordinary people who are still alive and who are willing for their writings to be studied in this way and to be questioned themselves as well.

The principal requirement is identification of a match between the material that is available and the empirical or theoretical question to be addressed. Perhaps this method is particularly appropriate for the lone individual, who can make him or herself expert in aspects of a particular person's life. The method is not only appropriate to theory testing by means of content analysis, using a system of defined categories, as in the examples cited. It could also be possible to apply a more qualitative, for example grounded theory, approach to identify the key themes in a person's account of an episode of development and/or adjustment in his or her life. The possibilities in fact are numerous. To practise in this field one does not even have to negotiate access to a fresh source of archive material. One can make use of the many available published collections of correspondence and diary accounts that do exist written by famous people. It is surprising that they are so little used by psychologists.

What is less easy to obtain is funding. Opportunities from external grant funding are likely to be limited for the foreseeable future. Writing about people in the public eye, of course, is a growth industry. But the royalties from writing books about famous people make investing time in writing about the non-famous even less attractive. Perhaps there are opportunities for such proposals to be fitted into more general research programmes where the topic fits. The important issue is to identify the value of the data source. Certainly there are plenty of opportunities here for postgraduate and even undergraduate projects.

Case study 2: *Self and identity in advanced old age*

In Erikson's theory the self is transformed in midlife through the development of 'generativity', the capacity to give to the next generation. In old age, the key issue according to the original theory is 'integrity', the acceptance of the gift of one's life. But what happens after the achievement of integrity? Erikson's reference to a 'post-narcissistic' approach to life implies the attainment of a certain kind of distance on one's history and the process of making it. There are problems, however, with this model of ageing. Since the theory was first formulated in the immediate postwar years increased numbers and higher life expectancy, accompanied by a decline in the average size of families and increase in the number of co-existing generations, has meant that the life experiences of older people nowadays are very different from those of their grandparents and even their parents (Jerrome 1993). From the standpoint of Erikson's theory, it can appear that many elderly people live on long after having apparently completed their life's story. What then is to be their purpose in living? This is a question that Erik Erikson and his wife Joan considered, as they became older themselves and wondered about a further ninth stage beyond that of 'integrity–despair' (Erikson 1998).

McAdams, who has perhaps done most in recent years to develop Erikson's theory of adult development, suggests that older people may finally move beyond story making, from making life meaningful through narrative. Desperate clinging to an identity rooted in the past does not appear ideal. Having accepted the gift of their life persons may come instead to live from day to day. Rather than being seen negatively as a regression to childhood, this may indicate a transcendence of history, a living in the 'eternal moment'. A number of recent gerontological authors refer to the possibilities of a shift from a materialistic–rational to a transcendent perspective on self and life in old age. For example, the concept of 'gerotranscendence' is used by Tornstam to refer to a shift in metaperspective, from a materialistic and pragmatic view of the world to a more cosmic and transcendent one

(Tornstam 1993). Joan Erikson draws on Tornstam's work in developing her own ideas (Erikson 1998).

This is only one perspective on the self in advanced old age. In our case study examination published in the *Journal of Personality* (Coleman *et al.* 1999) we considered this theoretical perspective alongside that related to management of self-esteem. The latter also draws a distinction between the earlier stages of ageing and the experience of growing frailty (Atchley 1991). Adjustment to the latter is more demanding and involves the right balance of 'immunizing' (e.g. denial, selective attention to evidence), 'assimilative' (e.g. self-correction and compensation) and 'accommodative' processes (e.g. rearrangement of priorities, rescaling of self-evaluative criteria) (Brandstadter and Greve 1994). All have their part to play, and skill is required in judging when one or the other is appropriate. However, in late life in particular, as energy levels fall, accommodative coping becomes more adaptive. According to Brandstadter and Greve, it is the failure to accommodate that more often marks depression at this stage of life.

Thus both perspectives imply that late life is marked by a different attitude to the self, that transcends personal history making and the previous criteria by which the self has been judged. As part of the completion of a 20-year longitudinal study of ageing, we decided to look at all the material we had collected related to the self on the surviving cases from our sample, and to compose case studies on them. The data available to us included not only questionnaire responses, but also interview transcripts and written self-descriptions obtained at different points in time. Following the methods advocated by Bromley (1977, 1986) we provided reasoned arguments in each case to account for change and stability in self-esteem and identity over the course of the study. The principal conclusions reached were presented to the participants for their comment and approval (Coleman *et al.* 1998).

In a subsequent analysis we decided to examine in particular detail the application of the two theoretical perspectives that I have outlined to a selected number of cases. We decided to choose the cases on the basis of the different types of 'self-trajectory' we had observed over the course of the study, i.e. those who had maintained consistent high self-esteem, those whose self-esteem had remained low throughout, those whose self-esteem had declined but then recovered, those whose self-esteem had shown more than one fluctuation, and those whose self-esteem had declined right at the end of life. For each category we selected a case on the basis of optimal representation of the particular trajectory type, the principle of 'prototypicality', an important criterion for deciding the appropriateness of a particular case for examination (Bromley 1986). Thus we chose 'Mrs Darby' to represent the group with consistent high self-esteem because she was the oldest member and because she had coped successfully with the largest number of life changes during the study. We reasoned that the resulting five cases we scrutinized should provide sufficient variety of material to test the explanatory power of the theories at the level of the individual case.

In our published description of this study (Coleman *et al.* 1999) we provided accounts of each person's history, followed by evidence relating to the application first of the management of self-esteem perspective and second of the identity as story perspective. Did these five people show the positive benefits of transcending the old self and the negative consequences of not doing so as they became more frail?

Although we found evidence for lack of accommodation coinciding with depressive episodes in some cases, as argued by Brandstadter, in general we did not find a clear distinction between processes of adjustment observed in earlier and later old age. Assimilative coping strategies continued to be used successfully, for example by Mrs Darby into her late nineties, attending as many social gatherings as she could. She had shown remarkable ingenuity in overcoming obstacles and re-establishing former goals, even managing to leave residential care for sheltered accommodation at the age of 92 years. The best example of accommodation is shown by 'Mrs Tinker' who has the lowest self-esteem but who is also not depressed. However, in her case it appears accommodation and low self-esteem have marked her whole life, which has been curtailed by circumstances beyond her control: her mother's frailty, her need to stay by her, and her husband's death after a short and greatly delayed marriage. She describes her life as limited but one to which she has adapted.

Similarly personal story telling does not appear to decline in importance in advanced old age. Partly this may be explainable in terms of our growing intimacy with the people we were studying, but not entirely. Story continues to be used not only in making sense of the past, but interpreting the present as well. In our meetings with Mrs Darby over the last years of her life she appears even more engaged in life review, exorcizing the ghosts of an unhappy childhood and explaining a subsequent marriage in terms of her wish to care for the man's children, and her dream now in her late nineties to meet the children in the homes for which she has been making soft toys. Also, Mrs Tinker appears to have become more reflective about the lack of control in her early life. This has helped her to set more realistic goals for the present.

Thus our close scrutiny of five 'prototypical' cases shows the relevance of concepts used in the literature to explain management of self-esteem and identity as story. But it does not provide support for the distinction being drawn between earlier and later old age. Continuity of process is more evident than discontinuity. Similar modes of coping have been demonstrated throughout the study, as people passed through their seventies to their eighties and even to their nineties. 'Mr Peck', for example, provides an example of a person who has struggled against the odds to preserve his desired style of life until the age of 90, who has suffered bouts of depression as a consequence, but who is now learning to accept what previously was unacceptable. But the accommodation is late coming, partial and somewhat grudging in character. More in-depth study is recommended into such exemplar cases of late life changes in ways of coping as a way of developing theory in this area. A combination of idiographic and nomothetic research is likely to produce more fruitful results than relying solely on the latter.

In addition, our study shows that it is eminently feasible to carry out such longitudinal case study analysis as part of a larger quantitative study. It requires additional resources but these can be built in at the outset of the planning of the project. The additional benefit can be justified in terms of the depth of understanding obtained. A subject as complex as the self requires a variety of approaches including case studies in which the person's own voice can be heard. If case studies are being used to validate theoretical concepts, the approach we have taken of selecting 'representative' or 'prototypical' cases seems an important principle to adopt. The method seems especially appropriate to research questions touching on human adjustment, such as bereavement, relocation and onset of frailty/disability.

There are practical limitations to the application of this method. One needs to be able to collect multiple sources of evidence about the individual involved (possibly including evidence from other observers as well) to justify the quasi-judicial approach and a strict approach to corroboration of evidence. In our study we relied on the variety of evidence from questionnaires, open interviews, and written accounts the participants sent to us through the post.

It is also important to bear in mind the personal requirements of such research. It is necessary in regard to each case studied for the investigator to have the ability and capacity, in terms of time and effort, to develop a relationship with the person concerned and to sustain it over a period of time, since it is unlikely that a worthwhile case study can be constructed from one or two interviews alone. It should also be remembered that the participants will need to give consent not only to the original investigation but also at a later stage to publication of the details of their lives in anonymized form. This makes it important to involve them in the final stage of written analysis, even if only at the level of major conclusions.

Conclusion

Psychological case studies are legitimate research activities which contribute to theory development but also fulfil one of the main aims of psychology, which is to understand the individual person. The field of ageing research provides good opportunities for such study in terms of availability of material and willingness of older people's involvement. Case analyses can be built into more general research proposals. One can distinguish between the use of case studies to investigate a person or issue about that person and its use to validate and develop existing theory by testing the theory's adequacy at the individual level. The latter use has been a major focus of the present chapter, and has closer parallels with hypothesis testing in nomothetic research. But case studies can also be used to explore a new or little understood phenomenon and to develop new theory about it. Case-law can be developed inductively on the basis of multiple cases drawn from the same population.

It is also possible for a community of researchers to work usefully on the same set of questions or problems, provided that they agree some common definitions and standards of methodology to be applied to the cases they study (Edwards 1998). Placing case analyses on the Internet, which Fishman (1999) has proposed, would also encourage such shared activity among researchers and promote the development of a pragmatic psychology which addresses real-life problems and issues. However inter-institution competition and arguments over ownership of research material militate against such developments. It is significant that these weaknesses are less evident among gerontologists than other social scientists. As others too have suggested (Bromley 1986), ageing provides one arena where case study research could flourish in the twenty-first century.

References

Alexander, I.E. (1988) Personality, psychological assessment and psychobiography, *Journal of Personality*, 56: 265–94.

Alexander, I.E. (1990) *Personology. Method and Content in Personality Assessment and Psychobiography*. Durham, NC: Duke University Press.

Allport, G.W. (1937) *Personality: A Psychological Interpretation*. New York, NY: Holt.

Allport, G.W. (1965) *Letters from Jenny*. New York, NY: Harcourt, Brace and World.

Atchley, R.C. (1991) The influence of aging or frailty on perceptions and expressions of the self: theoretical and methodological issues, in J.E. Birren, J.E. Lubben, J.C. Rowe and D.E. Deutchman (eds) *The Concept and Measurement of Quality of Life in the Frail Elderly*, pp. 207–25. London: Sage Publications.

Barlow, D.H. and Hersen, M. (1984) *Single Case Experimental Designs: Strategies for Studying Behavior Change*, 2nd edn. New York, NY: Pergamon Press.

Bate, W.J. (1977) *Samuel Johnson*. New York, NY: Harcourt Brace Jovanovich.

Boswell, J. ([1791] 1968) *The Life of Samuel Johnson*. London: The Folio Society.

Brandstadter, J. and Greve, W. (1994) The aging self: stabilizing and protective processes, *Developmental Review*, 14: 52–80.

Bromley, D.B. (1977) *Personality Description in Ordinary Language*. London: Wiley.

Bromley, D.B. (1986) *The Case-study Method in Psychology and Related Disciplines*. Chichester: Wiley.

Bromley, D.B. (1990) Academic contributions to psychological counselling: 1. A philosophy of science for the study of individual cases, *Counselling Psychology Quarterly*, 3: 299–308.

Bromley, D.B. (1991) Academic contributions to psychological counselling: 1. Discourse analysis and the formulation of case reports, *Counselling Psychology Quarterly*, 4: 74–89.

Coleman, P.G., Ivani-Chalian, C. and Robinson, M. (1998) The story continues: persistence of life themes in old age, *Ageing and Society*, 18: 389–419.

Coleman, P.G., Ivani-Chalian, C. and Robinson, M. (1999) Self and identity in advanced old age: validation of theory through longitudinal case analysis, *Journal of Personality*, 67: 819–49.

Edwards, D.J.A. (1998) Types of case study work: a conceptual framework for case-based research, *Journal of Humanistic Psychology*, 38: 36–70.

Elms, A.C. (1988) Freud as Leonardo: why the first psychobiography went wrong, *Journal of Personality*, 56: 19–40.

Erikson, E.H. (1958) *Young Man Luther*. New York, NY: Norton.

Erikson, E.H. (1963) Childhood and Society, 2nd edn. New York, NY: Norton.

Erikson, E.H. (1969) *Gandhi's Truth*. New York, NY: Norton.

Erikson, E.H. (1998) *The Life Cycle Completed* (extended version with new chapters on the ninth stage by Joan M. Erikson). New York, NY: Norton.

Fishman, D.B. (1999) *The Case for Pragmatic Psychology*. New York, NY: New York University Press.

Franz, C.E. (1995) A quantitative case study of longitudinal changes in identity, intimacy and generativity, *Journal of Personality*, 63: 27–46.

Freeman, M. (1993) *Rewriting the Self: History, Memory, Narrative*. London: Routledge.

Freeman, M. (1997) Death, narrative integrity, and the radical challenge of self-understanding: a reading of Tolstoy's *Death of Ivan Ilych*, *Ageing and Society*, 17: 373–98.

Freeman, M. and Robinson, R.E. (1990) The development within: an alternative approach to the study of lives, *New Ideas in Psychology*, 8: 53–72.

Hartley, J.F. (1994) Case studies in organizational research, in C. Cassell, and G. Symon (eds) *Qualitative Methods in Organizational Research*, pp. 208–29. London: Sage Publications.

Head, J. (1994) In memoriam: Erik Erikson 1902–1994, *The Psychologist*, 7: 325.

Jerrome, D. (1993) Intimate relationships, in J. Bond, P. Coleman and S. Peace (eds) *Ageing in Society: An Introduction to Social Gerontology*, 2nd edn, pp. 226–54. London: Sage Publications.

Keen, J. and Packwood, T. (1995) Case study evaluation, *British Medical Journal*, 311: 444–6.

Levy, L. (1970) Conceptions of Personality. New York, NY: Random House.

McAdams, D.P. (1988) Biography, narrative and lives: an introduction to the special issue on psychobiography and life narratives, *Journal of Personality*, 56: 1–18.

McAdams, D.P. and West, S.G. (1997) Introduction to special issue: personality psychology and the case study, *Journal of Personality*, 65: 757–83.

Mack, J.E. (1976) *A Prince of Our Disorder: The Life of T.E. Lawrence*. London: Weidenfeld and Nicolson.

Morgan, C.D. and Murray, H.A. (1935) A method for investigating fantasies, *Archives of Neurology and Psychiatry*, 34: 289–306.

Murray, H.A. (1938) *Explorations in Personality*. New York, NY: Oxford University Press.

Peterson, Bill E. and Stewart, A.J. (1990) Using personal and fictional documents to assess psychosocial development: a case study of Vera Brittain's generativity, *Psychology and Aging*, 5: 400–11.

Runyan, W.M. (1981) Why did Van Gogh cut off his ear? The problem of alternative explanations in psychobiography, *Journal of Personality and Social Psychology*, 40: 1070–7.

Runyan, W.M. (1984) *Life Histories and Psychobiography: Explorations in Theory and Method*. New York, NY: Oxford University Press.

Runyan, W.M. (1988) Progress in psychobiography, *Journal of Personality*, 56: 295–326.

Runyan, W.M. (1990) Individual lives and the structure of personality psychology, in A.I. Rabin, R.A. Zucker, R.A. Emmons, and S. Frank (eds) *Studying Persons and Lives*, pp. 10–40. New York, NY: Springer.

Runyan, W.M. (1997) Studying lives: psychobiography and the conceptual structure of personality psychology, in R. Hogan, J. Johnson and S. Briggs (eds) *Handbook of Personality Psychology*, pp. 41–69. San Diego, CA: Academic Press.

Shapiro, M.B. (1966) The single case in clinical psychological research, *Journal of General Psychology*, 74: 3–23.

Sisman, A. (2000) *Boswell's Presumptuous Task. Writing the Life of Dr Johnson*. London: Hamish Hamilton.

Stake, R.E. (1994) Case studies, in N.K. Denzin and Y.S. Lincoln (eds) *Handbook of Qualitative Research*, pp. 236–47. Thousand Oaks, CA: Sage Publications.

Steptoe, A., Reivich, K. and Seligman, M.E.P. (1993) Composing Mozart's personality, *The Psychologist*, February, 69–71.

Stewart, A.J. and Healy, J.M. Jr (1989) Linking individual development and social changes, *American Psychologist*, 44: 30–42.

Stewart, A.J., Franz, C. and Layton, L. (1988) The changing self: using personal documents to study lives, *Journal of Personality*, 56: 41–74.

Tornstam, L. (1993) Gerotranscendence – a theoretical and empirical exploration, in L.E. Thomas and S.A. Eisenhandler (eds) *Aging and the Religious Dimension*, pp. 203–25. Westport, CT: Greenwood Publishing Group.

White, R.W. (1952) Lives in Progress. New York, NY: Holt, Rinehart and Winston.

White, R.W. (1966) Lives in Progress, 2nd edn. New York, NY: Holt, Rinehart and Winston.

White, R.W. (1975) *Lives in Progress*, 3rd edn. New York, NY: Holt, Rinehart and Winston.

Yin, R.J. (1984) *Case Study Research. Design and Methods*. Beverly Hills, CA: Sage Publications.

10

Doing diary-based research

Bill Bytheway
Julia Johnson

Introduction

Research that focuses on 'everyday life' has to relate to questions of 'what happens in reality'. The challenge that gerontologists face is how to obtain, interpret and analyse data that is specifically about changes, events and actions that occur in the course of life. In our opinion, research into such concerns as 'activities of daily living' and 'the quality of life' should draw on the systematic study of day-to-day living and not just on retrospective in-depth interviewing. Interviews, of course, can be highly revealing about perceptions of past and present activities (Atkinson and Silverman 1997). In regard to a repeated action, for example, one can ask such questions as 'How often do you do it?' and 'When did you first start?' But, without the aid of relevant documentation, the response to such questions constitutes only a *retrospective account*, one that is totally dependent upon the interviewee's recall and interpretations of the question (Dingwall 1997). It is often argued that this is valid since it provides a subjective account of what is, or was, important to the interviewee as he or she sees it now. This is fine if the subjective perspective is what is being researched, but not if the subject of research is what happens in the course of everyday life.

Personal diaries are kept by many people as an aid and a supplement to memory. With an accumulating series of annual diaries, for example, they are able to return to past experiences and 'relive' them. No longer dependent solely upon memory, they can reflect upon and consider how they came to do what they did, and to be where they are now. In this way researchers are often urged to keep diaries and so it is logical to explore the wider possibilities of using diaries in research.

In this chapter we first review the potential of *commissioned* diaries as a tool for ageing research, and then report what we have learned from the use of one in a study of long-term medication and older people.

Definition of key terms

Diaries are documents that are made up of *fixed-length spaces* referenced to a consecutive series of *fixed-length time units* (Symes 1999). Entries are made as and when appropriate, often as part of the repeated routine of the time unit. A commercially produced diary, for example, may offer you one page for each day for a specific year, and at the end of every day you detail what you have done. But the time unit may be of any length, an hour or a week perhaps, and the *period* covered may be of any length too. Each time unit has an identifier, either a *date* or a *number,* and each diary an author, the *diarist.* It is important to distinguish diaries from other ways of recording events. For example, visits to a doctor can be entered in a personal medical record. Letters may be exchanged between friends. What distinguishes diaries from such logs and memoirs is the fact that a page, or some other fixed amount of space, is allocated *in advance* for every successive unit of time in the specific period.

Personal diaries are used by the diarist, retrospectively and prospectively, either as a simple source of basic information (appointments, etc.) or as a detailed and unfolding narrative. Diarists are free to use the diary for whatever purpose, making entries as and whenever they choose.

A *commissioned diary* is designed to obtain particular kinds of information for a specific research purpose. The *researcher* asks the diarist to keep it and offers appropriate instructions. It is a kind of self-completion questionnaire, covering any period and using any time unit. The same kinds of information are sought about each time unit throughout the period, and this is recorded according to a specific routine.

Plummer contrasts three broad strategies in the use of commissioned diaries (1983: 19–20). With an *unstructured* diary subjects are asked to think of it as an ordinary personal diary. The *time-budget* diary is intended to record how much time is spent on specific activities and when. With the *diary/interview* method, the diary is used as an aide-mémoire, a device that ensures that interviews relate to the interviewee's experience and not the researcher's presumptions.

Range of practice in this field

Throughout the twentieth century there was a continuing research interest in what diaries revealed about ordinary life.[1] Nevertheless when, in 1983,

Plummer undertook his exhaustive review of the use of documents by sociologists, he concluded that there had been 'remarkably little' use of diaries (1983: 18). There are certain areas of social research where diaries have been used extensively in the study of time use: for example, work and leisure (Sullivan and Gershuny 2001), and health service use (Rogers and Nicolaas 1998).

In regard to later life, Young and Schuller (1991: 107), following the lead of Townsend (1957: 296–313), have used individual diaries to illustrate extreme contrasts in post-work lifestyles. But some who have reviewed time use research in gerontology have been critical. Rubinstein and Moss (2000), for example, have noted that mainstream gerontology has been 'less than enthusiastic' about time use studies, and Powell Lawton (1999) has noted an emphasis on analysing variations between different groups (gender, living arrangement, income). Similarly, in regard to food and nutrition, Dickinson (1999) has noted an emphasis upon quantitative analysis of diaries.

In planning our research, we found two, very different, studies particularly helpful. Zimmerman and Wieder adopted the diary/interview method in studying counter-culture. They argued that, combined with the information resulting from an interview, the diary 'affords at least the possibility of gaining some degree of access to naturally occurring sequences of activity, as well as raising pertinent questions about their meaning and significance' (Zimmerman and Wieder 1975: 485). There is in this claim an interest both in what actually happens and in what this means. There is also recognition that research with such objectives is potentially fruitful but not easy.

The continuing UK Family Expenditure Survey (FES), the second study, uses a 14-day diary as a way of reducing reliance upon memory in recording household expenditure (Office for National Statistics 1999). As an adult in a sampled household you are requested to record 'everything which you yourself pay for', no matter how small and no matter when the goods might be delivered or obtained. Drawing upon evidence from this and related surveys, Kemsley (1979) identified various sources of bias. First, over a two-week period, more entries are made in the first few days than later in the week or in the following week. Second, the narrower the focus of the diary, the greater the likelihood of an event being recorded: when the diary recorded only one area of expenditure for example, spending in that area then appeared to be higher. Third, diary record keeping appeared to affect behaviour. A proportion of respondents in the FES admitted that they spent less when the diary had made them aware of what they were doing. Fourth, there was a differential response rate. For example, households where the head was retired were less likely to respond. The composition of the group willing to complete diaries, Kemsley concluded, could not be considered representative of the original sampled population (see also Lee 1993: 116).

Case study

Aims

Between 1998 and 1999 we undertook a study of how people aged 75 or more manage their long-term medication.[2] This was funded by the Department of Health and, not surprisingly, was linked to health service concerns with compliance. Fortuitously, at the same time, the Royal Pharmaceutical Society was promoting the concept of concordance: the idea that doctor and patient are engaged in an equal and collaborative alliance in which each respects the concerns, expertise and experience of the other. Reflecting this, the aim of our project was to see how older people manage their long-term prescribed medication and how they fit this into their everyday lives, and not just to examine how health service personnel attempt to achieve compliance.

The process

The method of recruiting participants is described in detail in Johnson and Bytheway (2001). Our objective was to obtain a representative sample of people aged 75 or over, who had been taking prescribed medication for 12 months or more and who were not in long-term residential, nursing or hospital care. Altogether a total of 133 eligible people were approached and 77 agreed to take part. For the fieldwork (in four contrasting areas of England and Wales) we recruited graduates who had experience of social science fieldwork but no professional training in health care or medicines.

The project's information leaflet explained the purpose of the research and how it would be conducted: participants being interviewed several times, showing the fieldworker their medicines and how they were stored, keeping a 14-day diary, and agreeing to the research team having access to their medical records. In the leaflet we indicated that participants were free to decline any of these requests and to drop out at any point.

In designing the diary, we decided that it should cover two weeks: anything longer might be too demanding for the participant. Anything shorter and we would risk not obtaining at least one uninterrupted and full week of diary entries.[3]

The diary was produced as an A4 size document. As Figure 10.1 shows, each of the fourteen days is represented by a double-page spread with a 6×24 grid, each of the 24 columns representing one hour. The rows related to six aspects of daily living. First, the consumption of medication had to be recorded. Next, we wanted to set medication into a broader context and so symptoms and meals were also included. Finally, phone calls, visitors and visits/shopping often affect and are affected by symptoms, meals and

Day 1

Date _____ *Notes*

_____ day

		Midnight 12	1	2	3	4	5	6	7	Morning 8	9	10	11	Midday 12	1	2	Afternoon 3	4	5	6	7	Evening 8	9	10	11	Midnight 12
1	Medicines taken																									
2	Symptoms felt																									
3	Meals or snacks																									
4	Phone calls																									
5	Visitors																									
6	Visiting or shopping																									

Figure 10.1 A typical diary two-page spread

medication and so these three aspects were also included. The grid occupied the middle third of each spread; the remainder was left blank for diarists to enter notes and other pertinent information. In this way, we created a structure to assist the diarists to produce a record of how medication fitted into their daily lives.

The following instructions were included on the front of the diary. They indicate how we endeavoured to create a diary-keeping routine and how we planned to make use of the diary in structuring the interviews:

> Think of this as an ordinary diary. There are fourteen pages, one page for each day of the fortnight. We have divided the day up into hours, and we have given you boxes to tick and a space at the top and bottom for you to make notes.
>
> According to the time, we want you to tick a box whenever:
> 1 you take your medicines
> 2 you feel symptoms or pains
> 3 you have a meal or snack
> 4 you have or make a phone call
> 5 visitors call
> 6 you go out visiting or shopping.
>
> When we come back to check the diary, we would like to ask you about these things. We are specially interested in when you take your medicines and whether anything out of the ordinary upsets your routines.
>
> So *whenever you tick a box, make a note* of what the symptom was, what medicines you took, who visited you, or whatever. Just enough to help you remember.
>
> Try to fill the diary in whenever it's convenient. At some point each morning, you should think back over the previous twelve hours and check that the diary is up-to-date. Likewise you should do the same in the evening.
>
> We hope you find this an interesting – or even helpful – exercise. We will keep in touch with you during the fortnight and will come to collect the diary when it is over. Many thanks for your help.

We piloted the diary with six participants. This led to a number of improvements in the design. More significantly, we became aware that some participants needed help in getting the diary started. It was important that the fieldworkers adopted the same strategy in relation to handing over and explaining the diary. Diarists were recruited and assisted as follows.

In the first interview, the fieldworker explained that, although we would like participants to complete the diary and to complete it themselves, this was not essential. If they wished, they could have the help of 'a scribe'. The diarist (participant or scribe) was then given the diary and shown how to complete it. Through our pilot study we had found that it was simplest to go back to 'this time yesterday' and then, with the participant, to begin making appropriate entries for the following 24 hours. In this way, most of the entries for Days 1 and 2 were made by the fieldworker. This was done with the participant providing information and the fieldworker showing how entries should be made. The fieldworker checked that the diarist understood the grid and then suggested ways of making notes. Thus, in most instances, Day 3 was the first day in the diary to be filled in solely by the diarist. At some point during the following interview, a few days later, the fieldworker looked over the diary, and may have added notes about actions that had not been recorded. If the diarist was having difficulty, the fieldworker would again use the procedure of going back over the previous 24 hours. On the final visit, prior to the diary being handed over, the fieldworker made sure it was completed as fully as possible.

Findings

The data that the diary generated were subjected to systematic analysis (Bytheway *et al.* 2000: 91–119). There were 64 participants for whom there were entries for at least seven days in the dairy. From these 64 diaries we transferred all records of medication on to charts that we called 'Medigrams'. It was not difficult to develop a typology which sorted the Medigrams according to the number of times in the day when medicines were con-sumed and the regularity of consumption. We then selected illustrative examples of each of these types and related their diary records to the kinds of medication being taken; to their lifestyles and their ways of managing their medication; and to the use of healthcare services (Bytheway *et al.* 2000: 98–110).

Figure 10.2 provides one example, the Medigram for Miss Neal.[4] She was one of 13 participants with a regular routine of medication twice a day that had been disrupted during the course of the fortnight. The following is a summary of what we learned about her medication:

> In interview, Miss Neal described how she takes her medicines rou-tinely at around 8 a.m. or 9 a.m. in the morning and again at 9 p.m. or 10 p.m. in the evening. In between times she goes out most days. Looking at her diary, we find that routinely she applies drops to her eyes when washing before breakfast. During the first week she then had a blood pressure tablet after breakfast. In the early hours of Day 5, however, she made a note of 'pain in neck and head'. This pain woke her again at 4 a.m. on Day 9. She went to see her doctor after break-fast, who changed her medicine and gave her a new prescription of lisinopril for her blood pressure problem. She took her first tablet that evening and continued taking it at the same time over the following days. She had noted on Day 1 that she always has Shredded Wheat,

Hr	Day 1	2	3	4	5	6	7	8	9	10	11	12	13	14	Total
1															
2															
3												c			1
4									c						1
5															
6															
7															
8		b	b	b	b	b	b	b	b	b	b	b	b	b	13
9	a	a	a	a	a	a	a	a	a			c			10
10					c					c			c		3
11														c	1
12															
13															
14															
15															
16															
17															
18															
19															
20											c				1
21	c	c	c	c	c	c			d	d			d		9
22							c	c	c	c	d	d	c	d	8
23														c	1
24															

a *Amlodopine Besylate 5mg (one daily)*
b *Viscotears Gel 10g (one drop as necessary)*
c *Co-codamol 8/500 (two up to four times a day)*
d *Lisinopril Dihydrate 2.5mg (one daily)*

Figure 10.2 The medigram for Miss Neal

tea and biscuits in the evening, and this had coincided during the first week with her taking co-codamol as a routine medication to control pain. In the second week, however, this pattern was unsettled. She also began to take co-codamol during the day and twice she took it at night to alleviate pain. Despite this health crisis, her basic routines were not changed and on Day 12, despite having taken the painkiller at 3 a.m., she went into town at midday to shop and have lunch out.

(Bytheway *et al.* 2000: 104)

This demonstrates well how a combined analysis of diary and interviews revealed a sequence of events associated with significant changes in prescribed medication and routines.[5] What this also offers is evidence of how medication relates to other aspects of daily life: washing, meals, social activities, symptoms of ill-health and use of health services.

Practical lessons

In Johnson and Bytheway (2001) we evaluated the diary with respect to five questions:

- *Representativeness*: to what extent did it put potential participants off, creating a sample more biased than would otherwise have been the case?
- *Difficulties*: were some participants unable to complete the diary due to visual impairment, problems of manual dexterity or limited literacy skills?
- *Quality of data*: how consistent, adequate and accurate was the diary as a record of daily events and actions?
- *Influencing behaviour*: did keeping a diary influence behaviour?
- *Ethical considerations*: did the completion of the diary, and all that went with it, cause undue distress, anxiety or inconvenience?

In the following, we summarize our conclusions about each of these in turn.

Representativeness

The information leaflet included a series of questions and answers about what we were asking of participants. On agreeing to take part, they signed a consent form and, in theory, knew that they would be asked to complete a diary, that this was not a requirement and that, if they wished, they could have the assistance of a relative or friend. Of the 133 eligible persons who were approached, 40.6 per cent refused to participate. We have some information about reasons for refusal, and none referred specifically to the diary. It became apparent, however, that not all those who agreed to take part had fully taken in the information in the leaflet and eight subsequently dropped out. Two said they were unwilling to keep the diary and this was the main reason for withdrawing from the project. The response of a third, Mrs Close, was more complicated, as indicated by the following report from the fieldworker:

> During the first interview, Mrs Close was happy talking about her health. However, when I started to explain the diary she became restless. She tried to talk more generally about her health and I would try and get her to talk more specifically about her day. When we had done the previous 24 hours she told me that she wasn't sure about the diary. I told her to fill in what she could but not to worry about it too much.

She still seemed unsure that she could do it and I then said that I would help her fill it in when I returned on my next visit. The next morning I received a phone call from Mrs Close. She said that she had been up most of the night worrying about the project and that she no longer wished to participate. I asked if it were the diary that she was worried about and she said that she didn't know. I then asked her if I could come back for my second visit anyway and that she should leave the diary. She told me I could come if I wanted to. I visited Mrs Close for a second time. She seemed surprised to see me at the door. I told her that she didn't have to do the diary, but it would help the project if I could talk to her again about her medicines. She said again that she didn't want to do the project. She gave me back the diary (with only the one day filled in that I had completed with her) and the patient information leaflet. I was surprised that Mrs Close dropped out in this way as she had seemed such a willing participant in the beginning. It is most likely that the diary had put her off but I have wondered too whether her niece or nephew had advised her against her participation.

This account illustrates well both the anxiety that a request to participate in intensive research can generate, and the problems of obtaining an explanation for refusals and dropouts.

We concluded that among those who refused to participate or who subsequently dropped out, there were two linked anxieties about the diary. The first was that of exhibiting a 'lack of competence': completing the diary appeared to be a test of both literacy and the ability to follow instructions. The second was that the written record could, in some unknown way, be used against them: they were not taking their medicines 'as instructed' and were afraid the doctor would 'find out'. They were unconvinced by our assurances of complete confidentiality. In contrast, some may have been keen to participate, perhaps to show how good they were in complying with the doctor's orders. Short of a control group, however, we are not able to test for such biases.

The wide variety both of approaches to completing the diary and – on the evidence of the diary – to medicine taking suggest that these were not strong tendencies and that the sample was 'reasonably representative'. We estimated that between 5 and 10 per cent of those invited to participate had misgivings about the diary which subsequently led to them refusing or dropping out. This may be less than might be expected, particularly for this age group. Nevertheless, they may have been some of the more interesting and significant members of the sample and, in this sense, their absence will have introduced an important element of bias.

Difficulties

We were concerned that those who would have difficulties in completing the diary, due to poor vision, dexterity, comprehension or literacy, should not be excluded, nor feel excluded, and so the information leaflet indicated that they were free to recruit 'a scribe'. From our final sample of 77, we received 56 fully completed diaries (defined as diaries that had entries – of any kind – on at least 13 days).[6] Of these, nine were completed by a scribe: three daughters, three wives, one husband and two fieldworkers. These participants needed help due to poor sight or arthritis, and in five instances their medication was routinely managed by the scribe.

Twelve of the 47 participants who kept their own diaries said they had difficulties. Also, of the ten who started but did not complete their diaries, there were five who found the task too difficult due to specific illnesses or impairments. Although such difficulties led to some incompleteness and inconsistency, they also served to illuminate some of the problems that participants and carers face in managing medication.

Quality of data

Some participants who had no difficulty in making entries still produced incomplete diaries. The fieldworkers were instructed to check the diaries and, on a few occasions, they challenged participants over the completeness of the record. For example, Mrs Austin insisted that she took one Trental tablet three times a day 'with or just after food'. Despite this, her diary record indicated that, although she always took one with her breakfast, there were five days when she missed her lunchtime tablet and seven when she missed the one with the evening meal. The fieldworker subsequently commented:

> Mrs Austin told me she 'always makes a point of taking these' [Trental]. However, looking through the diary on my second visit [on Day 7], I noticed that she had not taken her third tablet on several evenings – as she had been out unexpectedly with friends. When I mentioned these omissions to her, she told me that she 'must carry some spare in her handbag'. When I mentioned this again on my third visit [on Day 18], Mrs Austin insisted that she never on any occasion misses taking her Trental.

Mrs Austin felt embarrassed by these inconsistencies, and the fieldworker did not press her into checking and correcting the diary. As a result we are left, for example, guessing that she took her evening Trental on Days 2, 3 and 6: that it was the diary, not her tablets, that she had neglected. Whatever the case, this evidence conveys something of the problems entailed in thrice daily medication for people with a busy social life.

Another concern about the quality of the data was that there would be a *decline in the detail* recorded. We investigated this by counting the words used in making notes (Johnson and Bytheway 2001). There was a decline during the first week from an average of 41.0 words on Day 3 to 33.4 words on Day 7, but no further decline during the second week.

In the large majority of cases, the participants followed the instructions they were given (see above). A particular event or activity was noted – in the diarist's own words – and linked to a ticked box indicating both a subject and a time of day. This, we feel, is the real strength of the design: with a minimum of effort, the diarist was able to provide us with a detailed and chronologically specific account of the events of the day.

Nevertheless, there were some minor complications. Seven diarists were poor at *linking* ticks and notes, particularly for busy or complicated days. Four attempted to resolve this by entering *codes* into the boxes to indicate the medicines they took. Some entered extravagant ticks covering several boxes. When an activity took up more than one hour (e.g. shopping), three participants ticked all the relevant boxes and four others drew a line through the boxes. Similarly six participants had symptoms that were experienced constantly and they wrote a description of these through the boxes in the row marked 'Symptoms', sometimes covering the whole day. These inadequacies in the design of the diary did not seriously reduce the quality of the information obtained. Rather they reflect some of the un-certainties that our diarists faced in summarizing and symbolizing their day on the two-page spread.

Most limited their entries to the six subjects we had specified and did not record other aspects of their day. Many were convinced that they led highly routine lives. Even though the fieldworker had pointed out that there were two pages at the end of the diary to record the usual daily and weekly routines, six entered comments on the diary pages such as 'My routine is the same nearly every day' (Mr Garlick, Day 5). Given this, when nothing actually disturbed the routine, the diarist must have been tempted to take short cuts. For example, 18 entered a term such as 'usual tablets' on at least one day. Although we do not know from this what was actually taken, interviews with these diarists indicated that such en-tries represent several tablets being taken in a single act, sometimes having been placed in a dish by a carer. In this way the diary/interview method provides important insights into the management and consumption of multiple medication.

We suggested that diarists made entries in their diaries every twelve hours (see above). Despite this, some may not have followed this routine. One of our fieldworkers, for example, noted that in one diary the entry for the whole of the day of her second visit had already been filled in before she arrived. Were there others who similarly knew in advance what they were going to do? The diary of Mr Kirk appears to fit in with this scenario. There are two clues. First, on each of Days 3 to 14 he wrote '7 a.m.: Get up' (note that he did not write '7 a.m.: Got up'). Second, next to this, on each of the ten weekdays of his fortnight, he wrote the following words: '8.15 a.m.: Warden buzzed me on the intercom to ask if I was alright'. Despite its length, exactly the same wording was used on all ten days. Similarly all his various medicines were carefully written out in full detail on every page, and there is only one variation in either wording or timing: on the two Sundays, he recorded a trip out into the country which caused him to take his evening medication one hour later than usual. In contrast to these repetitive entries, he entered full details of his meals and social activities and no two days were the same.

Quite possibly, the warden did buzz him *every* weekday at 8.15 a.m. on the dot. But, equally, he may have sat down at some point and written the words out because he knew that this is what 'she always does' (and similarly entered his medicines on the same basis). The fieldworker's visits, however, are a check against this, and logs for visits to Mr Kirk on Days 4 and 8 include the notes: 'Diary: went through last few days', and 'Diary: checked over' respectively. This appears to confirm that Mr Kirk did write out his entries routinely every day.

We were also concerned that some of our participants, having described how their doctors had stressed the importance of following instructions for particular medicines, may have found it difficult to record any deviation in their diaries. Only a few diaries, however, were as unvarying as Mr Kirk's. There were many more who, we are sure, would have been embarrassed had the omissions and variations in their diaries been reviewed by their doctors.[7]

For the most part, the diaries exhibit a consistency and a level of specific and varying detail that suggest that they provide valid insights into actual days lived. In particular, they reveal much about how older people tailor their consumption of prescribed medicines in order to sustain their health and to suit their other routines and commitments.

Influencing behaviour

None of the diarists gave any indication that they specifically changed their routines or medication in the light of their diary keeping. At a relatively trivial level, diary keeping is bound to affect behaviour: no one makes diary entries mindlessly. At the very least, ticking for medicines taken is an action that can hardly be anything other than a check: 'Did I take it at lunchtime? Of course I did. I've ticked the box.' Indirectly, we actively encouraged participants to use the diary as a check when, in the information leaflet, we wrote: 'We hope you find this an interesting – or even helpful – exercise.'

Ethical considerations

Local Research Ethics Committees are concerned about the impact of research upon participants. In presenting our project for approval by the four committees covering our fieldwork areas, some misgivings were expressed that we were asking 'too much' of our participants. We countered this by stressing that participants were told they were free to drop out at any time and that they did not have to undertake all that we were asking of them. Partly because of these reassurances, eight dropped out before the concluding interview, three did not start a diary, and seven others ceased making diary entries before the end of the 14-day period.

Where participation in the study served to add a further strain on complex caring relationships, however, there were ethical issues to be addressed. A powerful illustration of this is provided by Mrs Ankers. Her diary was kept by her two daughters; initially by Ann, a nurse, who was visiting for a few days and then, after Day 10, by Joy, the daughter with whom Mrs Ankers lived. The fieldworker wrote:

> Her daughters were concerned about the amount of out-of-date medication that their mother had in the TESCO bag (under her bed). They told me they would dispose of it in the correct manner. I sensed this was a source of embarrassment to them – I did not ask to log any more medication which was left in the bag.

Obviously there is the potential here for Ann, the nurse, to suspect or accuse her sister of 'not looking after their mother properly'. At another point, Mrs Ankers embarrassed Joy by being rude about her GP ('I hate his bloody guts', she said). Joy tried to assure the fieldworker that 'her mother had no reason to feel this way about this doctor'. Thus participation in the research, including the production of the diary record, could have had a significant and potentially damaging impact upon relationships concerned with Mrs Ankers's care.

Different ethical issues were raised when, despite our assurances, some participants felt obliged to try to complete their diaries themselves even though they had real difficulties. As with any activity, it is hard to abandon a diary once started. There was the potential humiliation of being found incapable of completing it by the fieldworker.

Moreover, the whole business of recording daily life can be distressing if it reinforces the perception that one is leading an inactive, limited, dull or routine life, in sharp contrast perhaps to earlier years. Mrs Harper provided us with the clearest illustration of this reaction. She lived alone and had had a stroke. Nevertheless, she persisted with an active social life including amateur drama which she documented in her diary in tiny, scratchy writing. The diary, however, became too distressing for her and she gave it up after nine days. In her last entry she wrote:

> I find this too difficult and my head goes [indecipherable]. I realise that the record is no good unless it is accurate, and it gives a wrong impression. So reluctantly I feel I must decline to do any more and I apologise for wasting your time. I keep trying to improve and trying not to think about how having a stroke has changed my life and changing into a lesser something of the person I used to be. Doing this record over the last days has made me realise that I am chasing the 'moon' and it is quite impossible . . .

This example, more than any other, raised questions for us about the ethics of using diaries as a research tool. We had realized before we began that diary keeping (like reminiscence: see Coleman 1986) can be painful for some people, and this possibility had been discussed with the fieldworkers during our briefing meetings. No pressure was put on Mrs Harper by the fieldworker to continue (or on any of the others who gave up), and subsequently we wrote to thank her, reassuring her that her participation had been most valuable. Nevertheless we regret that she had felt obliged to make this long last entry.

The participant's collaboration with the fieldworker could be a positive experience. We were heartened, for example, by the following report by Miss Neal's fieldworker:

> She was quite troubled when I showed her the diary and how to fill it in . . . She had very poor eyesight and 'wobbly' handwriting, and felt that she would be unable to fill in the diary sufficiently. Much of the first visit was spent reassuring her, and going through the diary again and again until she felt comfortable. In the end, I feel that she did a wonderful job.

On Day 3, Miss Neal recorded 21 words and this increased to 34 on Day 14.

The only diarist who used the diary to produce a more general commentary on her situation was Mrs Tyrrell, acting as scribe for her husband. She said that they were both housebound. Her diary covered a fortnight dominated by four unconnected complications in their lives: changing the clocks to summer time, the closure of a local hospital (where their daughter worked), the death of Mr Tyrrell's sister (who had not left a will), and a crisis over renewing their own supplies of medication. On the last day, Mrs Tyrrell wrote that she had enjoyed doing the diary, and added the following acerbic (and somewhat disjointed) remarks:

> One thing I feel about Dr's visits – that something sometimes – that the GP could enquire how the 'Carers' are keeping fit & keep going all the time – very tired at times. Perhaps a tonic – not spirits?

Possibly she enjoyed participating because for once she was able to record her concerns herself, in her own words, and to describe some of the pressures under which she and her husband were living.

Further research

Through our evaluation we identified ways in which our use of the diary could have been improved. In analysing the diary data and the interviews we were often left uncertain about what had actually happened. Nevertheless, the diaries have revealed much about daily routines of medication and it is hard to know how else these kinds of insights could have been achieved. For this reason we think further research is warranted and we have a number of suggestions to make.

First, it is clear that more intensive work, with perhaps only a few subjects, would reveal much about the problems of adequately recording the events of a day. This should investigate the strengths and weaknesses of structured and open-ended formats and the potential sensitivities of older people embarking upon this task. Second, we would welcome a large-scale survey that investigated the extent of non-commissioned diary keeping among older people, and the potential of this for gerontological research. Several of our participants kept their own journals for a variety of purposes and, as with published memoirs, there is potentially much to be learnt from such documents. A third important area of research is the relationship between researcher and researched, and the benefits and costs of much more active forms of collaboration, or of payments being made to diarists.

Last, we would welcome comparable research to our own into other aspects of the daily lives of older people. Currently we are analysing the data we have collected on visits and visiting, and this is revealing a complex patterning of weekly routines and incidental contacts. In some cases where care professionals or paid carers were involved, there was a large number of people interacting in the participant's social world. For this reason, a detailed diary-based study of people receiving care services may test some of the models of community care which, to us, seem dangerously simplistic. For example, it is often assumed that the identity of 'the primary carer' will be apparent to service providers. Yet there was more than one participant whose diary revealed a much more complex pattern of support than that described in interview. Moreover, some of these participants were actively engaged in community life as well as receiving support. Research based on diaries would help to illuminate this neglected issue: the positive two-way relationship between community and older people.

On a more theoretical point, we would argue that current research into later life relies excessively on interviews with older people (Bytheway, forthcoming). This tends to underpin two popular ageist assumptions. The first is that old age is 'another world' and only by questioning 'the old' can we learn about its realities. The second is that, due to age, older people are not capable of participating in different and more challenging kinds of research. We would welcome more participative research, using methods such as the diary/interview, and we are confident that this will begin to challenge some of the more familiar conclusions of gerontological inquiries.

Funding sources

We suspect that there is a certain reluctance on the part of funders and their advisers to fund innovative research. It may be that the ethical issues entailed in investigating the lives of 'vulnerable' people in detail has counted against such proposals. Or it may be that funders are unwilling to challenge the acquiescent functionalism that still characterizes much social research in this area (Townsend 1981).

It is certainly the case that practitioner research using methods such as the diary/interview would entail close collaboration and, straying into matters of assessment, this would raise some delicate ethical issues. Nevertheless we are confident that if such research were to be seen as a genuine collaboration between practitioner and user, these matters could be resolved.

Current developments regarding participative research[8] suggest that we should be anticipating gerontological research both being commissioned (and perhaps funded) by agencies managed by older people themselves, and being undertaken by older researchers. Undoubtedly the diaries of such researchers will become an increasingly valuable source of insight into later life and so it seems probable that the diary/interview method will become increasingly central to gerontological research.

Conclusion

Overall, we have concluded that, for gerontological research, the diary/ interview method:

- can provide extremely detailed over-time data;
- can greatly reduce the problem of accurate recall;
- can set specific actions (such as medication) in the broader context of everyday events;
- can help to distinguish what people *actually* do from what they *say* they do;
- can offer insights into many aspects of daily living in later life: eating, drinking, sleeping, dressing, washing, cleaning, repairing, travelling, shopping, reading, writing, telephones, television, internet, singing, dancing, etc.

In planning the use of diaries in gerontological research, our advice would be to keep it simple, to offer the diarists clear instructions and lots of space, to spend time with them getting it started, and to check regularly on progress, asking, at the same time, questions about what has been happening and what is being recorded. Potentially it is a great way of doing research *with* older people.

The diary has provided us with the opportunity to reflect on the power and significance of the handwritten word: research subjects are producing a record 'by hand', 'in their own words' and 'in their own time'. Some of our participants appreciated that what is expressed 'in writing' is of much greater social significance than what might be said in passing, and most were concerned that what was recorded was accurate. In a material sense, this was 'their account'.

In three of the diaries there is the handwriting of someone other than the diarist or fieldworker. There is an expression of trust implicit in the fact that the participant allowed this to happen. As in the appointment of scribes, such entries reflect a close involvement in the participant's daily life. So here, in the written word itself, we have evidence of support for the participant. There is a striking contrast to such evidence in Miss Neal's diary. Close to two ticks in the 3 a.m. column for Day 12 (see Figure 10.2), there is an entry, written in wobbly writing, recording a headache and the taking of a co-codamol tablet. Of course we cannot be sure when she made this entry, but there is a visual power in this lonely image of pain in the middle of the night that could never be conveyed by other research methods.

Notes

1 See Ponsonby (1923); Allport (1942); Fothergill (1974); Verbrugge (1985); Coxon (1988); Wheeler and Reis (1991); Berman (1994); Elliott (1997); Gershuny and Sullivan (1998); and Bell (1998).
2 This study, *The Management of Long-term Medication by Older People* was undertaken between April 1997 and June 1999 and was funded by the Department of Health (Bytheway *et al.* 2000).
3 The Family Expenditure Survey has considered various time periods and undertaken 'experiments'. It concluded that 14 days is the best 'compromise solution' (Kemsley *et al.* 1980: 36). The two-week diary is still being used by the FES (Office for National Statistics 1999: 156).
4 The names used in this paper are the same as those used in Bytheway *et al.* (2000). All are pseudonyms.
5 We were subsequently able to check this account further against Miss Neal's medical record kept in her GP's practice.
6 One diary was collected on the fourteenth day, before the participant had made any entries. Another two participants inadvertently turned two pages and so made entries for only 13 days.
7 In the Information Leaflet, participants were assured that neither the doctors nor any other member of the primary care team would have access to the tapes or transcripts of the interviews.
8 See Peace (1999); Carter and Beresford (2000); Hayden and Boaz (2000); and Warren and Maltby (2000).

References

Allport, G.W. (1942) *The Use of Personal Documents in Psychological Science*. New York, NY: Social Science Research Council.
Atkinson, P. and Silverman, D. (1997) Kundera's immortality: the interview society and the invention of self, *Qualitative Inquiry*, 3(3): 324–45.

Bell, L. (1998) Public and private meanings in diaries: researching family and childcare, in J. Ribbens and R. Edwards (eds) *Feminist Dilemmas in Qualitative Research*. London: Sage Publications.

Berman, H. (1994) *Interpreting the Aging Self: Personal Journals of Later Life*. New York, NY: Springer Publishing.

Bytheway, B. (forthcoming) Positioning gerontology in an ageist world, in L. Andersson (ed.) *Cultural Gerontology*. Westport, CT: Greenwood.

Bytheway, B., Johnson, J.S., Heller, T. and Muston, R. (2000) *The Management of Long-term Medication by Older People. Report to the Department of Health*. Milton Keynes: The School of Health and Social Welfare, The Open University.

Carter, T. and Beresford, P. (2000) *Age and Change: Models of Involvement for Older People*. York: Joseph Rowntree Foundation.

Coleman, P. (1986) *Ageing and Reminiscence Processes: Social and Clinical Implications*. Chichester: John Wiley and Sons.

Coxon, T. (1988) Something sensational . . . The sexual diary as a tool for mapping detailed sexual behaviour, *Sociological Review*, 36: 353–67.

Dickinson, A. (1999) Food choice and eating habits of older people: A grounded theory. Unpublished PhD thesis, Buckinghamshire Chilterns University College, Brunel University.

Dingwall, R. (1997) Accounts, interviews and observations, in G. Miller and R. Dingwall (eds) *Context and Method in Qualitative Research*. London: Sage Publications.

Elliott, H. (1997) The use of diaries in sociological research. *Sociological Research Online*, 2(2), http://www.socresonline.org.uk/socresonline/2/2/7.html (accessed 27 June 2002).

Fothergill, R.A. (1974) *Private Chronicles: A Study of English Diaries*. Oxford: Oxford University Press.

Gershuny, J. and Sullivan, O. (1998) The sociological uses of time-use diary analysis, *European Sociological Review*, 14(1): 69–86.

Hayden, C. and Boaz, A. (2000) *Making a Difference*. Better Government for Older People Evaluation Report. Coventry: Local Government Centre, University of Warwick.

Johnson, J.S. and Bytheway, B. (2001) An evaluation of the use of diaries in a study of medication in later life, *International Journal of Social Research Methodology*, 4(3): 183–204.

Kemsley, W.F.F. (1979) Collecting data on economic flow variables using interviews and record keeping, in L. Moss and H. Goldstein (eds) *The Recall Method in Social Surveys*, Studies in Education No. 9, pp. 115–41. London: University of London Institute of Education.

Kemsley, W.F.F., Redpath, P.U. and Holmes, M. (1980) *Family Expenditure Survey Handbook*. London: HMSO.

Lee, R.M. (1993) *Doing Research on Sensitive Topics*. London: Sage Publications.

Office for National Statistics (1999) *Family Spending: A Report on the 1998–99 Family Expenditure Survey*. London: The Stationery Office.

Peace, S.M. (ed.) (1999) *Involving Older People in Research: 'An Amateur Doing the Work of a Professional?'* London: Centre for Policy on Ageing/Centre for Ageing and Biographical Studies.

Plummer, K. (1983) *Documents of Life*. London: George Allen and Unwin.

Ponsonby, A. (1923) *English Diaries*. London: Methuen.

Powell Lawton, M. (1999) Methods and concepts for time-budget research on elders, in W.E. Pentland and A.S. Harvey (eds) *Time Use Research in the Social Sciences*. New York, NY: Kluwer Academic/Plenum Publishers.

Rogers, A. and Nicolaas, G. (1998) Understanding the patterns and processes of primary care use: a combined quantitative and qualitative approach, *Sociological Research Online*, 3(4), http://www.socresonline.org.uk/socresonline/2/2/7.html (accessed 27 June 2002).

Rubinstein, R.L. and Moss, M. (2000) *The Many Dimensions of Aging*. New York, NY: Springer.

Sullivan, O. and Gershuny, J. (2001) Cross-national changes in time-use: some sociological (hi) stories re-examined, *British Journal of Sociology*, 52(2): 331–48.

Symes, C. (1999) Chronicles of labour: a discourse analysis of diaries, *Time and Society*, 8(2): 357–80.

Townsend, P. (1957) *The Family Life of Old People*. London: Pelican.

Townsend, P. (1981) The structured dependency of the elderly: a creation of social policy in the twentieth century, *Ageing and Society*, 1(1): 5–28.

Verbrugge, L.M. (1985) Triggers of symptoms and health care, *Social Science and Medicine*, 20: 855–70.

Warren, L. and Maltby, T. (2000) Averil Osborn and participatory research, in A.M. Warnes, L. Warren and M. Nolan (eds) *Care Services for Later Life*. London: Jessica Kingsley Publishers.

Wheeler, L. and Reis, H.T. (1991) Self-recording of everyday life events: origins, types and uses, *Journal of Personality*, 59(3): 339–54.

Young, M. and Schuller, T. (1991) *Life after Work: The Arrival of the Ageless Society*. London: HarperCollins.

Zimmerman, D.H. and Wieder, D.L. (1975) The diary-interview method, *Urban Life*, 5(4): 479–97.

11

Doing evaluation of health and social care interventions

Ann Netten

Introduction

While many older people are fit and lead active lives, as a group older people are major consumers of health and social care services. Clearly it is important that such services are delivered effectively and efficiently. But in order to achieve this we need evidence about how well current services and policies are doing, how they can be improved and the resources needed.

There is an increasing demand for 'evidence-based' practice, particularly in the fields of health (National Institute for Clinical Excellence 1999) and social care (Department of Health 2000). This 'evidence base' depends fundamentally on the results of evaluative research. The classic definition of evaluation is 'a method for determining the degree to which a programme meets its planned objective' (Suchman 1967). Others have argued that this defines evaluation too narrowly. Robson (1993) argues that it is only, at best, a part of what evaluation might concern itself with. Other issues would include unintended consequences, the importance of context, and understanding of the mechanisms by which the programme generates (or is hypothesized to generate) outcomes (Pawson and Tilley 1997). Ideally, good quality evaluative research identifies what works, why, in what circumstances, and, if it is an economic evaluation, at what cost.

There is no attempt to be comprehensive in descriptions of approaches to evaluation here: there are whole libraries of books and learned societies devoted to evaluation. The objective is simply to provide some context and a critical appraisal of a particular approach to evaluation of health and social care interventions, based on the Production of Welfare theoretical framework. This framework has been applied in a variety of contexts, but primarily to evaluations of health and social care interventions for older people, an area often neglected in evaluative research. The study presented is an exemplar of how theoretical principles inform design.

Approaches to evaluation

Over two decades ago Patton (1981) estimated that there were over 100 different approaches and they have certainly multiplied since. These arise, *inter alia*, from differences in their philosophical base, objectives and perspectives.

Philosophical base

The two principal philosophical approaches are the *positivist* approach, which usually is associated with quantitative research, and the *phenomenological* approach, more often associated with qualitative research. Positivism is the basis of the natural sciences, which have the aim of discovering laws using experimental and quantitative methods, with the emphasis on facts. Phenomenology emphasizes that social 'facts' are characterized by their meaningfulness to members of the social world.

The difference can be exemplified by the role of theory within each approach (see Box 11.1). A positivist approach uses theory as a basis for identifying hypotheses to be tested and questions that need to be asked. Most economic evaluations are based in the positivist approach. Phenomenological social scientists argue that research observation precedes theory and the aim is to discover social meanings (Bowling 1997). For example, 'grounded' theory develops during the course of an investigation with the investigator feeding back and testing emerging findings (Glaser and Strauss 1967).

The objectives of an evaluation can be classified in terms of the use to which the research is to be put and the focus and scope of the evaluation (see Box 11.2). Formative evaluations collect data during a programme or intervention, or about an organization while it is active, with the aim of developing or improving it. Summative evaluation involves collecting data about the programme, intervention or organization either during or after with the aim of deciding whether it should be continued or repeated (Kemm and Booth 1992).

In terms of the scope of an evaluation Donabedian (1980) distinguishes three key aspects of any intervention that will be of concern to evaluators: structure, process, and outcome. Structure refers to the organizational framework, process to the activities undertaken, and outcome to the consequences of those activities such as the numbers and qualifications of people involved

Box 11.1   Types of research question

Positivist

- Have policy incentives to maintain people in their own homes resulted in an increased level of impairment and dependency in care homes? What are the cost implications of rising levels of impairment and dependency in care homes (Netten *et al.* 2001)?
- What is the expected length of stay of older people after admission and what influences this (Bebbington *et al.* 2001)?

Phenomenological

- What is the importance of home and independence to older people (Means 1998)?
- How do older people feel about independence and involvement? How do their lives embody the ideas and values associated with these two concepts (Abbot and Fisk 1997)?

Box 11.2   Types of evaluation research

Formative

- Quality assurance exercises in care homes (see for example Centre for Environmental and Social Studies in Ageing 1992; Kellaher and Peace 1993).

Summative

- Investigation of the reality of user involvement in care planning and the extent to which choice is exercised (Myers and MacDonald 1996).
- Evaluation of the effectiveness of community care of older people (Bauld *et al.* 2000).

in the training or service. The objective of the formative evaluations would be to identify problems and successes in the process of introducing training and accreditation procedures or the specialist service. The summative evaluation would focus on the effect of the training or service on outcomes for older people. Process information would inform the findings about success or otherwise of the innovations.

In their Realistic Evaluation approach, Pawson and Tilley (1997) would add context and mechanism to this list. In addition to spatial and institutional locations (factors that could be described as structure), context encompasses the norms, values and interrelationships found within them. Mechanisms refer to the choices and capacities that lead to regular patterns of social behaviour. These are relevant both to the causes of the problem to be addressed by the intervention and the way in which it is anticipated that an intervention is expected to have the desired effect. In our examples context would include the regimes of the homes and aspirations and motivations of staff. Mechanisms would include theories about how the training, specialist regimes and advice services were expected to impact upon competence and behaviour.

Perspectives

Necessarily there will be a variety of perspectives on the programme, intervention or policy to be evaluated. These can include, for example, users of services, carers of users of services, care staff, service provider or purchaser, 'expert', government and society. The positivist approach emphasizes the importance of a detached 'objective' assessment. Pluralism aims to take on board a variety of perspectives using approaches such as triangulation, which uses different methods and sources of information to address specific aspects of interventions (Kellaher 1990). In our examples in Box 11.2 the perspectives of staff and residents might be gained through questionnaire, interview and direct observation. Economic evaluation emphasizes the importance of the societal perspective in estimating costs and outcomes. Much emphasis is put on identifying the benefits to individuals (both residents and staff) and society's valuation of these benefits.

Involving users in the design and conduct of evaluative research is increasingly important to funders and is discussed elsewhere in this volume (cf. Chapter 14). It has also been argued that to engage the motivation of participants the evaluation approach has to be consistent with the principles and contribute to the purpose of the activity being evaluated (Barr and Hasagen 2000).

Requirements of evaluation

Different forms of evaluation have their particular strengths and weaknesses, so it is important to tailor the approach to the particular situation and the requirements of funders and other potential users of the findings.

In practice qualitative approaches, based in the phenomenological tradition, are essential for exploring new topics and obtaining insights into complex issues. These are more often used in formative evaluations and often focus on process issues and identifying the different perspectives of stakeholders: older people, their carers, paid direct care and professional staff, managers and policy makers. Quantitative techniques, usually based in the positivist tradition, are appropriate if the issue is known about, relatively unambiguous and amenable to valid and reliable measurement (Bowling 1997). These are more often used in summative projects and tend to be more focused on structure and outcome than process.

As Challis and Darton (1990) point out, the term evaluation implies using criteria to make a judgement about the effectiveness or success of a policy or intervention. In order to identify whether an intervention has had the desired effect it is important to have a point of comparison. This can be against agreed criteria for success, for example expert judgement, before and after the intervention takes place, or against a comparison group.

Particularly in the health field there is an emphasis on demonstrating causality (or that the study has *internal validity*) through experimental approaches such as randomized controlled trials (RCTs). In RCTs people are randomly allocated to two or more groups that are subject to different treatments or interventions. Because they are randomly assigned, any systematic effect of other factors should be eliminated. The argument is often made that this is the best way to demonstrate the effects of an intervention. It is most prevalent in the field of medical and health service research where it is often referred to as the 'gold standard' (Bowling 1997).

However, there are problems with this type of approach. For example, it is important in such designs to undertake power calculations in order to make sure the sample size is large enough to detect a true difference (see Bland 1995 for the method and formula). In some instances the sample size required may be too large to be achievable, either because of the lack of suitable subjects (for example, a problem when considering older service users from ethnic minorities) or because the expected variation in the effect to be measured is so large. The latter is often the case when demonstrating cost-effectiveness is the object of the exercise (Gardiner *et al.* 2000). Moreover, by randomizing the effects that might affect costs and outcomes the design eliminates the very factors that may be of interest in more complex types of intervention. Such factors might include the effect of age, gender, the role of informal carers and living circumstances on outcomes for older people. Although stratified samples can be used to control for expected effects and thus used to estimate the size of these effects, there are limits to how many such groups are practical.

An important issue for users of research, particularly those concerned with implementing 'evidence-based' policies and practice, is the generalizability of results. The problem with in-depth qualitative research is that, while providing fresh insights, it cannot demonstrate how widely applicable the findings are. The problem with purely experimental methods is that they create artificial situations that may not apply in the 'real world', so have limited *external validity*. Such studies are vulnerable to the 'Hawthorne effect', where people change in some way as a result of the research process (Roethlisberger *et al.* 1939). The problem with evaluations of interventions in natural settings is distinguishing effects due to the intervention rather than other contextual or unmeasured factors. Experimental designs such as RCTs allocate subjects such that other influences should apply equally to each group, so there is no need to measure or take into consideration these factors.

RCTs work well when there is a clearly defined and controllable intervention, such as the introduction of a new medication or physical therapy. However, in many health and social care situations the effect of the intervention depends crucially upon the process, which may vary according to the characteristics and circumstances of the individuals concerned. For example, the success of the care management process for older people depends on the complexity of need-related circumstances, availability of different service options and attitudes and expectations of those involved (Challis and Davies 1986). Approaches such as the one described here and Realistic Evaluation (Pawson and Tilley 1997) investigate in depth what works for whom and in what circumstances. While this can be combined with the experimental method, there is a greater emphasis on understanding the process, range of effects and mechanisms at work.

The approach that we are discussing here is based in the positivist tradition, using theory as a basis for identifying the issues to be addressed and questions to be asked. The theoretical framework is called the Production of Welfare.

Production of Welfare (PoW)

The Production of Welfare (Davies and Knapp 1981; Knapp 1984) has its roots in economics and was developed primarily for the social care context. In the field of health care evaluation a sophisticated body of knowledge has built upon health economics, a discipline increasingly called on as funders of research demand information about costs and cost-effectiveness in addition to evaluations of the effectiveness of interventions (see Drummond *et al.* 1997 for a valuable guide to the principles of health economic evaluations).

Figure 11.1 illustrates the PoW framework, which seeks to identify the relationship between resources, needs and outcomes. In this approach the ultimate outcome, the welfare of individuals, is represented as the result of a combination of inputs. Resource inputs include staff time, capital (such as buildings) and consumables (such as heating and travel costs). These are combined in the form of services that can be measured as units of output: home care hours, residential care weeks and so on. The impact of these resources on outcomes will be influenced by intangible inputs, which include the characteristics of service users and attitudes of care staff. The role of

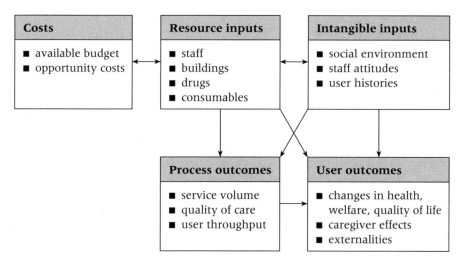

Figure 11.1   Production of Welfare

informal carers can similarly be divided between resource and intangible inputs. A further development of the framework, the Social Production of Welfare, puts the informal care network at the heart of the production process and represents services as an input to the household of the service user (Netten and Davies 1990).

The PoW framework draws on economics, so has a positivist starting point. However, as we shall see, in application it is characterized by a broader, pluralistic, multidisciplinary approach. In contrast, health economic evaluations are often associated with clinical trials, so adopt an approach closer to the natural sciences.

In order to illustrate the issues that need to be taken into consideration when designing and conducting an evaluation using the PoW framework we turn to specific studies that have put this into practice.

Evaluation in practice

All PoW evaluations to date have been summative, prospectively evaluating experiments or current practice. They have been widely acclaimed as examples of good practice and as influential on community care policy (Griffiths 1988; Department of Health 1989, 1993).

Examples of PoW studies

Perhaps the best known of the evaluations that have been conducted using this approach are the Care Management experiments (Challis and Davies

1986; Davies and Challis 1986; Challis *et al.* 1990, 1997). These were all evaluations of an (at the time) innovative approach to managing and organizing care for very frail or dependent older people. The framework was also used as the basis for an evaluation of the 1980s policy of discharging long-stay hospital patients into community settings. The Care in the Community project evaluated 28 demonstration projects in which people from a variety of client groups were discharged into a range of community-based settings throughout England and Wales (Renshaw *et al.* 1988; Knapp *et al.* 1992). The long-term implications of this policy continue to be evaluated through a series of follow-up studies (Cambridge *et al.* 1994). In addition to prospective evaluations of experiments or new policies, the approach has been used to evaluate mainstream community care (Davies *et al.* 1990; Bauld *et al.* 2000; Davies *et al.* 2000).

Here we focus on the evaluation of the Darlington project (Challis *et al.* 1995), which was one element of the Care in the Community programme. The project had five objectives:

- to maintain at home a group of physically disabled older people who would otherwise have remained in long-term hospital care;
- to introduce trained home care assistants to cover tasks that would have previously been undertaken separately by health and social care workers;
- to provide a higher quality of care and satisfaction among project service users and their families than they would have experienced had they been in hospital or receiving mainstream community care services;
- the cost of providing home care was to compare favourably with long-stay hospital care; and
- the service was to provide an additional level of long-term care in the community for frail older people living in the area.

This was to be achieved through the introduction of a model of care that involved care management and coordination at four levels: between agencies, through multidisciplinary working, individual care management and the trained care worker (Challis *et al.* 1995).

The objectives of the evaluation were to:

- examine how appropriate the community care model was for patients with varying degrees of physical and mental frailty;
- compare the effects of community care with those of institutional care on family and other informal carers;
- compare the relative costs of care at home and long-stay hospital care; and
- examine whether health and social services were effectively integrated at the individual client level (Challis *et al.* 1995).

Thus the evaluation was addressing both care process and cost and effectiveness issues. The underlying objective was to identify the characteristics of patients for whom discharge from hospital and the provision of non-institutional forms of long-term care were most appropriate and represented the best use of resources. It is this type of information that is most useful for users of research when considering the generalizability of the findings.

Design

A key aspect of the evaluation was to demonstrate causality: to identify whether the community care model was more effective than, or at least as effective as, institutional care in caring for people. This suggests the need for an experimental approach. Challis and Darton (1990) discuss the issues that need to be taken into consideration in experimental designs in this type of context in some detail. Here we just focus on the issue of random allocation, as the RCT was described above as the 'gold standard' in health care evaluations for demonstrating causality.

A number of factors were taken into account when deciding against a random allocation in Darlington (Challis *et al.* 1995). These factors apply to a wide range of health and social care evaluations and include:

- resistance among service providers which might result in the design being sabotaged;
- political unacceptability of appearing to deny to some people a new service seen as potentially better for clients;
- potential for contamination, for example by reducing workload in the comparison service so changing the amount of time practitioners have available to spend with and on clients; and
- a randomized experiment can provide evidence about whether an intervention produces a particular change rather than why the result occurred. One of the key research questions was how applicable the care model was, a question that requires a wider collection of information, including process issues.

As a result a *quasi-experimental* method was used (Campbell and Stanley 1966). In this, people receiving the intervention are compared with a group who have similar characteristics. Such comparison groups can be drawn from waiting lists for the intervention, in an area where the intervention has not been implemented or in the same area before the implementation of the intervention. In the Darlington study the comparison groups were drawn from an adjacent health district.

The intervention and comparison groups were assessed in hospital and followed up six months later. A census of older patients that was conducted in both health districts before the intervention allowed a comparison to be made, with potential for matching cases on an individual basis. In addition, to allow a comparison with mainstream community services, a sample of older people who attended day hospital and their carers were interviewed. Again, sample size is important in such designs, although it is often, as in this study, dictated by the capacity of the intervention. All 101 older people who were discharged from hospital as part of the three-year funded intervention were recruited into the intervention group. The comparison groups were based on 113 people who remained in hospital and 30 older people using the day hospital. It was possible to identify and interview 75 carers of older people in the intervention group, 27 carers for the hospital comparison group, and 30 for the day hospital group.

Measurement

Identifying the information required is usually undertaken through self-completion questionnaires or structured or semi-structured interviews. It is important to pilot the approach before undertaking the main fieldwork in order to ensure reasonable response rates and identify misunderstandings or problems in practice that could lead to poor quality data at a later stage.

Costs and inputs

One of the distinguishing characteristics of the PoW framework is the emphasis that is put on the measurement and effect of resource inputs. The cost of these inputs provides a basic building block to any subsequent analysis of the relationship between needs, resources and outcomes. Netten and Beecham (1993) bring together the theoretical background and practical guidance to the estimation and use of cost information.

The estimated cost depends on the perspective: society, public expenditure, an individual agency or private individual. Ideally, the perspective is that of society so all the resource consequences of an innovation or policy are identified. However, for certain purposes there may be more interest in a specific perspective such as the implications for the public purse or to an agency, such as social services. In the Darlington study the costs were estimated and analysed from a variety of perspectives: society, social and health care agencies, and community service costs.

Costs are measured through identifying the level of resources used and valuing these resources by multiplying them by their unit cost. In the Darlington study resources used were recorded on a weekly basis by project staff. This was used to provide information about the flow of resources to each client for six months following discharge from hospital. The Client Service Receipt Inventory (Beecham 1995) has been developed, which provides a useful framework for the collection of resource use data. However, this is not a 'one size fits all' approach and has to be adapted to reflect the needs of individual projects. Unit costs are ideally based on local information, but for those resources infrequently used, or where information is difficult to acquire, a series of volumes, *Unit Costs of Health and Social Care*, is helpful (see 'Resources', page 191). It is essential in using such sources to ensure that the unit cost is appropriate to the way the resources have been measured.

In undertaking or evaluating the costing element of an evaluation, four costing 'rules' are helpful (Knapp 1993):

- *Costs should be comprehensively and accurately measured.* In the Darlington study local information about unit costs was used and resource use, including expenditure by carers, was carefully monitored and tracked over time. Where assumptions had to be made sensitivity analyses were undertaken to identify the impact of these on estimates made, and thus potentially on conclusions drawn.
- *It is important to reflect and explore variations.* In the Darlington study information was collected at an individual level enabling multivariate analyses of factors associated with costs from a variety of perspectives.
- *Like should be compared with like.* The quasi-experimental design helped ensure that like was compared with like. It was also important that living expenses were estimated for those living in the community as such costs are included in hospital costs. The simple measurement of care package costs would underestimate resource use of care in the community.
- *Cost information should be linked with outcomes.* A key aspect of the Darlington evaluation was to compare outcomes between those discharged into the community and those who remained in hospital. The approach to this is discussed below.

One particular aspect of the opportunity cost that the study did not address was the opportunity cost of the time of informal carers. Both measuring and attributing a value to informal care is the subject of considerable debate (Netten 1993; Smith and Wright 1994; Posnett and Jan 1996; Brouwer 1999).

Intangible inputs

The relevant intangible inputs to any particular intervention are context-specific. In the Darlington study these included the needs or dependency of individuals, the social networks on which they could draw, and the type of help provided by the informal carer.

In the measurement of intangible inputs and outcomes it is important to ensure validity (that the measure is measuring what you want it to measure) and reliability (that the same measurement would result from the same circumstances regardless of who administered the instrument or when it was administered). This is best achieved by using established scales that have been tested for these properties. The more widely the measures have been used in other evaluations, the more the particular characteristics of individuals or effects of interventions can be compared and set in context. It is also important to ensure that the scales are appropriate and address issues relevant to older people.

In the Darlington study a wide variety of standard scales were used to reflect the characteristics of the older people and their carers including the Behaviour Rating Scale from the Clifton Assessment Procedures for the Elderly (Pattie and Gilleard 1979), which was used to measure dependency, and the Interview Schedule for Social Interaction (Henderson *et al.* 1981), to measure social networks.

Several measures were based on previous work or scales, adapted to be applicable and relevant to older people, and questions used in previous studies. Although such measures and questions did not have demonstrated validity and reliability they benefited from the practical development and application of the instrument on which they were based. For example, the Social Behaviour Assessment Scale (SBAS) that had been designed to estimate the burden of care of people caring for acute psychiatric patients (Platt *et al.* 1980) was adapted to be applicable for carers of older people.

When designing an evaluation it is important to consider carefully what it is you want to measure and to investigate the literature to identify whether others have developed appropriate instruments. Since the time the Darlington study was being designed there has been a proliferation of scales (e.g. Wenger 1994, 1997) and some advice on measurement (Royal College of Physicians and British Geriatrics Society 1992a, 1992b; Department of Health 2001a). Wilkin and Thompson (1989) and Wilkin *et al.* (1992) also provide useful information about measurement of needs and outcomes in health care. Bowling (1997) provides a very helpful guide to questionnaire and question design, including a description of the types of scales that are used for identifying attitudes and views. Quantitative scales or indicators cannot capture all aspects of intangible inputs. In addition the care management process was monitored using structured case notes and regular reviews based on earlier studies (Challis and Chesterman 1985).

Process

An important dimension of the intervention was coordination and inter-agency working. Key to understanding the reasons behind success or failure of such initiatives is an analysis of the process. In the Darlington study information about the process was drawn from a number of sources:

- reports and minutes of meetings of the coordinating group, multidisciplinary groups and the project team who were organizing the intervention;
- notes kept by the project manager and the research worker;

- semi-structured interviews with care managers, home care assistants, and a wide range of professionals;
- diary sheets completed by home care workers and clients;
- case records including care plans.

Information was collected through the planning, implementation and consolidation stages of the project. This facilitated an understanding of why the project worked. For example, issues identified in the planning and pre-implementation phase included lack of clarity about boundaries of responsibilities and communication and liaison problems over admission and discharge. In the implementation phase multidisciplinary case conferences were identified as having an increasingly important role in coordinating assessments and care plans. In the consolidation phase improved relations were identified between hospital and community services.

Outcomes

A key characteristic of health and social care is the multiplicity of outcomes. This includes the types of outcomes and the people who benefit. In PoW the final or ultimate outcomes include the welfare or benefit to service users and their carers. Intermediate outcomes would include quality of care, type of care package and deferral of admission to residential care.

It is essential that the measure(s) selected to measure outcome should reflect the objectives of the intervention. In the Darlington study outcomes were measured in terms of destination: whether people were at home, in institutional care or had died, and change in quality of care and quality of life. This last was identified through change in subjective well-being, measuring changes over the six month period in levels of depression, using the General Health Questionnaire (GHQ) as a measure of depression (Goldberg 1972) and morale, using the Philadelphia Geriatric Morale Scale (PGMC) developed by Lawton (1975).

As the primary provider of care, the impact on informal carers is a key aspect of any evaluation of community care interventions. In the Darlington study, this was reflected through comparing scores of measures such as the Malaise Inventory to measure carer stress (Rutter *et al.* 1970), indicators of carer burden (based on the SBAS, see above) and the positive benefits of caring (Qureshi *et al.* 1983; Qureshi and Walker 1989). Rather than measuring change these scores were compared across the project and control groups.

Analysis

The design of the study will fundamentally affect the types of analysis that can be conducted. Experimental designs facilitate comparisons between groups. The PoW framework supports the use of cost and production function analysis, multivariate analyses used to explain variations in costs and outcomes respectively. Clearly multiple outcomes make production function analysis complex (Davies *et al.* 2000).

In the Darlington project outcomes were compared across the project and comparison groups. The groups were found to be so similar in terms of the initial characteristics that cases were not individually matched as had been originally planned, but compared using analysis of variance with statistical adjustments to reflect the minor differences (Challis and Darton 1990; Challis *et al.* 1995). This is a more efficient use of data as individual matching can result in lost data due to non-matches being found for some cases. Better outcomes were identified among those older people participating in the project in terms of destination, quality of care and well-being.

This then raised a number of questions: at what cost were these outcomes achieved; what affected outcomes; what was the implication for carers; and what were the important process lessons to be learnt? The comprehensive nature of the data collection allowed all of these issues to be explored in some depth. For example, weekly and total costs were found to be significantly lower for the project clients than for those remaining in hospital from the perspective of society, the public purse and care agencies. It was possible to explain 75 per cent of the variation in costs for project clients by indicators of the care process, health and dependency characteristics on discharge and informal care factors. This equation could then be used to predict the costs for the control group patients. The process data collected allowed a detailed description of the nature of the intervention and what aspects of it were most valued by older people and their carers, giving insight into the causal mechanisms at work.

Since the time of the study, and particularly in the field of health economics, statistical analysis, particularly of cost data, has advanced considerably (Barber and Thompson 1998; Chisholm 2000). This is important because cost distributions are often very skewed, with relatively few very high cost cases that need to be included as they represent real cost implications for the implementation of interventions and policies in practice.

Application of approach

This type of approach to evaluation is appropriate when there is a clearly identifiable intervention with hypothesized effects to be tested. The particular strength of comprehensive evaluations using the PoW framework is the identification of needs, resources and outcomes, answering the question of the type of person for whom the intervention is effective, in which contexts, and at what cost. As a result the studies using this approach have been very policy influential.

The weaknesses of the approach include the following.

- Such comprehensive evaluations are very resource intensive, requiring major research funding.
- To date there has been a lack of user involvement in the design of the research and identification of research questions.
- Unintended outcomes are not identified in a systematic way (a problem with all bar the most exploratory research approaches).

However, it is not always necessary to undertake both large-scale and in-depth studies when undertaking evaluations. Smaller scale studies are possible which a single researcher with limited resources can conduct. For example, a study of 13 homes focused on the effect of intangible inputs, in terms of the physical and social environment, on older people with dementia (Netten 1993). This used a before–after design on a sample of 10 residents from each home. The basic principles of such small-scale, more focused evaluations are similar to those described above, but necessarily there are limitations: the number of interviews that can be conducted being the most obvious.

Practical considerations

The Department of Health has published a helpful framework for the governance of research in health and social care which identifies the responsibilities of those who conduct, participate in, fund and manage health and social care research (Department of Health 2001b).

Important practical issues for those conducting research to bear in mind when planning health and social care evaluations are as follows.

- Clarify what the overall objectives of the evaluation are and develop hypotheses and a practical design that should allow these to be tested.
- Allow time to negotiate access. Social and health care professionals are protective of their clients and patients and will want to be clear that you are not going to waste their time.
- The MRC guidelines on good research practice require that the Local Research Ethics Committee, Multi-Centre Ethics Committee, or other appropriate ethics committee must approve all research involving identifiable personal information or anonymized data from the NHS.
- Should the study involve four or more local authority social services departments (SSDs), permission should ideally be sought from the Association of Directors of Social Services. This will increase the probability of SSDs participating. A fee is payable for this service.
- Pilot the overall research approach and individual questionnaires to identify misunderstandings and practical problems before undertaking the main evaluation.
- While facilities such as care homes and day centres provide a captive audience, they are often over-researched.

- Respect people's privacy and desire not to participate.
- When deciding on the initial sample size remember that response rates are a function of the characteristics of the population being studied.
- Postal questionnaires can increase numbers but there tend to be more response rate problems.
- Volunteer, and remember, to feed back results to those participating in the research.

Summary

- There is a wide variety of approaches to evaluation; the most appropriate approach will depend to an extent on the research question.
- The experimental method, one example of which is the RCT, is powerful in attributing causality but has limitations when the interest is in what works for whom in what circumstances.
- The PoW framework, which is set in the positivist economic tradition, brings together key aspects of needs resources and outcomes and their relationships. In practice evaluations based on this framework have tended to take a comprehensive approach, beyond that usually adopted in economic evaluations in other fields.
- This type of approach is helpful, and policy influential when addressing clearly defined interventions/services.
- Comprehensive evaluations of needs resources and outcomes are resource-intensive. However, it is possible to investigate more focused aspects of the production of welfare on a more limited scale. Such studies are more likely to be limited in terms of their external validity.
- Engage critical faculties when evaluating other people's research.

Resources

Methods

Bowling, A. (1997) *Research Methods in Health: Investigating Health and Health Services*. Buckingham: Open University Press.
Drummond, M.F., Stoddart, G.L. and Torrance, G.W. (1997) *Methods for the Economic Evaluation of Health Care Programmes*. Oxford: Oxford City Press.
Huck, S.W. (2000) *Reading Statistics and Research*. New York, NY: Longman.

Measures

Royal College of Physicians and British Geriatrics Society (1992a) *High Quality Long-Term Care for Elderly People*. London: Royal College of Physicians.
Royal College of Physicians and British Geriatrics Society (1992b) *Standardised Assessment Scales for Elderly People*, London: RCP/BGS.

Wilkin, D., Hallam L. and Doggett, L. (1992) *Measuring Need and Outcome for Primary Health Care.* Oxford: Oxford University Press.

Costs

Netten, A. and Beecham, J. (1993) *Costing Community Care: Theory and Practice*, PSSRU Studies. Aldershot: Ashgate.
A series of volumes, annually published from 1993, *Unit Costs of Health and Social Care.* Canterbury: PSSRU University of Kent at Canterbury.

Acknowledgements

I am grateful to Robin Darton, David Challis and Katharine Netten for their helpful comments on earlier drafts of this chapter. Also to Judy Lee for her help in identifying useful websites.

References

Abbot, S. and Fisk, M. (1997) *Independence and Involvement: Older People Speaking.* St Albans: Abbeyfield Society.
Barber, J. and Thompson, S. (1998) Analysis and interpretation of cost data in randomised controlled trials: review of published studies, *British Medical Journal*, 317: 1195–200.
Barr, A. and Hasagen, S. (2000) *ABCD handbook: A Framework for Evaluating Community Development.* London: Community Development Foundation.
Bauld, L., Chesterman, J., Davies, B., Judge, K. and Mangalore, R. (2000) *Caring for Older People: An Assessment of Community Care in the 1990s.* Aldershot: Ashgate.
Bebbington, A., Darton, R. and Netten, A. (2001) *Care Homes for Older People. Volume 2: Admissions, Needs and Outcomes.* Canterbury: Personal Social Services Research Unit, University of Kent at Canterbury.
Beecham, J. (1995) *The Client Service Receipt Inventory*, Discussion Paper 1492/C053. Canterbury: Personal Social Services Research Unit, University of Kent at Canterbury.
Bland, M. (1995) *An Introduction to Medical Statistics.* Oxford: Oxford University Press.
Bowling, A. (1997) *Research Methods in Health: Investigating Health and Health Services.* Buckingham: Open University Press.
Brouwer, W.B.F. (1999) *Time and Time Costs in Economic Evaluation: Taking a Societal Perspective.* Ridderkerk: Ridderprint.
Cambridge, P., Hayes, L. and Knapp, M. (1994) *Care in the Community: Five Years On.* Canterbury: Personal Social Services Research Unit, University of Kent at Canterbury.
Campbell, D.T. and Stanley, J.C. (1966) *Experimental and Quasi-Experimental Designs for Research.* Chicago, IL: Rand McNally.
Centre for Environmental and Social Studies in Ageing (1992) *Inside Quality Assurance.* Newport Pagnell: IQA Consortium.

Challis, D. and Darton, R. (1990) Evaluation research and experiment in social gerontology, in S.M. Peace (ed.) *Researching Social Gerontology*. London: Sage Publications.

Challis, D., Chessum, R., Chesterman, J., Luckett, R. and Traske, K. (1990) *Case Management in Social and Health Care: The Gateshead Community Care Scheme*. Canterbury: Personal Social Services Research Unit, University of Kent at Canterbury.

Challis, D., Darton, R., Johnson, L., Stone, M. and Traske, K. (1995) *Care Management and Health Care of Older People: The Darlington Community Care Project*. Aldershot: Arena.

Challis, D., von Abendorff, R., Brown, P. and Chesterman, J. (1997) Dementia: challenges and new directions, in S. Hunter (ed.) *Research Highlights in Social Work 31*. London: Jessica Kingsley.

Challis, D.J. and Chesterman, J. (1985) A system for monitoring social work activity with the frail elderly, *British Journal of Social Work*, 15: 115–32.

Challis, D.J. and Davies, B.P. (1986) *Case Management in Community Care*. Aldershot: Gower.

Chisholm, D. (2000) 'Mind how you go': issues in the analysis of cost-effectiveness in mental health care, *Mental Health Research Review*, 7: 33–8.

Collin, C., Wade, D.T., Davies, S. and Horne, V. (1988) The Barthel ADL Index: a reliability study, *International Disability Studies*, 10(2): 61–3.

Davies, B. and Fernandez, J. with Nomer, B. (2000) *Equity and Efficiency Policy in Community Care: Needs, Service Productivities, Efficiences and their Implications*. Aldershot: Gower.

Davies, B.P. and Challis, D. (1986) *Matching Resources to Needs in Community Care: An Evaluated Demonstration of a Long-Term Care Model*, PSSRU Studies. Aldershot: Gower.

Davies, B.P., Bebbington, A. and Charnley, H. with Baines, B., Ferlie, E., Hughes, M. and Twigg, J. (1990) *Resources, Needs and Outcomes in Community-Based Care: A Comparative Study of the Production of Welfare for Elderly People in Ten Local Authorities in England and Wales*, PSSRU Studies. Aldershot: Gower.

Davies, B.P. and Knapp, M.R.J. (1981) *Old Peoples' Homes and the Production of Welfare*. London: Routledge and Kegan Paul.

Department of Health (1989) Cm 849, *Caring for People: Community Care in the Next Decade and Beyond*. London: HMSO.

Department of Health (1993) *Implementing Caring for People*, EL(93)18/CI(93)12. London: Department of Health.

Department of Health (2000) *A Quality Strategy For Social Care*. London: Department of Health.

Department of Health (2001a) *National Service Framework for Older People*. London: Department of Health.

Department of Health (2001b) *Research Governance Framework for Health and Social Care*. London: Department of Health.

Donabedian, A. (1980) *Explorations in Quality Assessment and Monitoring: The Definitions of Quality and Approaches to its Assessments*. Ann Arbor, MI: Health Administration Press.

Drummond, M.F., Stoddart, G.L. and Torrance, G.W. (1997) *Methods for the Economic Evaluation of Health Care Programmes*. Oxford: Oxford City Press.

Duncan, P.W., Wallace, D., Min Lai, S. *et al.* (1999) The Stroke Impact Scale Version 2.0: Evaluation of reliability, validity, and sensitivity to change, *Stroke*, 30: 2131–40.

Gardiner, J.C., Huebner, M., Jetton, J. and Bradley, C.J. (2000) Power and sample size assessments for tests of hypotheses on cost-effectiveness ratios, *Health Economics*, 9: 227–34.

Glaser, B. and Strauss, A. (1967) *The Discovery of Grounded Theory*. Chicago, IL: Aldine.

Goldberg, D.P. (1972) *The Detection of Psychiatric Illness by Questionnaire: A Technique for the Identification and Assessment of Non-Psychotic Psychiatric Illness*. London: Oxford University Press.

Griffiths, R. (1988) *Community Care: Agenda for Action*. London: HMSO.

Henderson, S., with Byrne, D.G. and Duncan-Jones, P. (1981) *Neurosis and the Social Environment*. Sydney: Academic Press.

Huck, S.W. (2000) *Reading Statistics and Research*. New York, NY: Longman.

Kellaher, L. and Peace, S. (1993) Rest assured: new moves in quality assurance for residential care, in J. Johnson and R. Slater (eds) *Ageing and Later Life*, 168–77. London: Sage Publications.

Kellaher, L., Peace, S. and Willcocks, D. (1990) Triangulating Data, in S. Peace (ed.) *Researching Social Gerontology*. London: Sage Publications.

Kemm, J.R. and Booth, D. (1992) *Promotion of Healthier Eating: How to Collect and Use Information for Planning, Monitoring and Evaluation*. London: HMSO.

Knapp, M. (1984) *The Economics of Social Care*. London: Macmillan.

Knapp, M. (1993) Principles of Applied Cost Research, in A. Netten and J. Beecham (eds) *Costing Community Care: Theory and Practice*. Aldershot: Ashgate.

Knapp, M.R.J., Cambridge, P., Thomason, C. *et al.* (1992) *Care in the Community: Challenge and Demonstration*. Gower: Ashgate.

Lawton, M. (1975) The Philadelphia Geriatric Center Morale Scale: a revision, *Journal of Gerontology*, 30: 85–9.

Means, R. (1998) Home, independence and community care: time for a wider vision, *Policy and Politics*, 25(4) 409–19.

Myers, F. and MacDonald, C. (1996) 'I was given options not choices', in R. Bland (ed.) *Developing Services for Older People and their Families*. London: Jessica Kingsley.

National Institute for Clinical Excellence (1999) *Appraisal of New and Existing Technologies: Interim Guidance for Manufacturers and Sponsors*. London: National Institute for Clinical Excellence.

Netten, A. (1993) Costing informal care, in A. Netten and J. Beecham (eds) *Costing Community Care*. Aldershot: Ashgate.

Netten, A. and Beecham, J. (eds) (1993) *Costing Community Care: Theory and Practice*, PSSRU Studies. Aldershot: Ashgate.

Netten, A. and Davies, B. (1990) The social production of welfare and consumption of social services, *Journal of Public Policy*, 10(3) 331–47.

Netten, A., Darton, R., Forder, J. and Bebbington, A. (2001) *Care Homes for Older People. Volume 1: Facilities, Residents and Costs*. Canterbury: Personal Social Services Research Unit, University of Kent at Canterbury.

Pattie, A. and Gilleard, C. (1979) *Manual of the Clifton Assessment Procedures for the Elderly*. Sevenoaks: Hodder and Stoughton.

Patton, M.Q. (1981) *Creative Evaluation*. Newbury Park and London: Sage Publications.

Pawson, R. and Tilley, N. (1997) *Realistic Evaluation*. London: Sage Publications.

Platt, S., Weyman, A., Hirsch, S. and Hewett, S. (1980) The Social Behaviour Assessment Schedule (SBAS): rationale, contents, scoring and reliability of a new interview schedule, *Social Psychiatry*, 15: 43–55.

Posnett, J. and Jan, S. (1996) Indirect cost in economic evaluation: the opportunity cost of unpaid inputs, *Health Economics*, 5: 13–23.

Qureshi, H. and Walker, A. (1989) *The Caring Relationship: Elderly People and their Families*. London: Macmillan.

Qureshi, H., Challis, D. and Davies, B. (1983) Motivation and rewards of helpers in Kent Community Care Scheme, Discussion Paper 0202/2. Canterbury: Personal Social Services Research Unit, University of Kent at Canterbury.

Renshaw, J., Hampson, R., Thomason, C. *et al.* (1988) *Care in the Community: The First Steps*. Aldershot: Gower.

Robson, C. (1993) *Real World Research: A Resource for Social Scientists and Practitioner-Researchers*. Oxford: Blackwell.

Roethlisberger, F.J. and Dickson, W.J. with Wright, H.A. (1939) *Management and the Worker: An Account of a Research Program Conducted by the Western Electric Company, Hawthorne Works, Chicago*. Cambridge, MA: Harvard University Press.

Royal College of Physicians and British Geriatrics Society (1992a) *High Quality Long-Term Care for Elderly People*. London: Royal College of Physicians.

Royal College of Physicians and British Geriatrics Society (1992b) *Standardised Assessment Scales for Elderly People*. London: RCP/BGS.

Rutter, M., Tizard, J. and Whitmore, K. (1970) *Education, Health and Behaviour*. London: Longman.

Smith, K. and Wright, K. (1994) Informal care and economic appraisal: a discussion of possible methodological approaches, *Health Economics*, 3: 137–48.

Suchman, E.A. (1967) *Evaluative Research*. New York, NY: Russell Sage Foundation.

Wenger, G.C. (1994) *Support Networks of Older People: A Guide for Practitioners*. University of Wales, Bangor: Centre for Social Policy Research and Development.

Wenger, G.C. (1997) Social networks and the prediction of elderly people at risk, *Aging and Mental Health*, 1(4): 311–20.

Wilkin, D. and Thompson, C. (1989) *User's Guide to Dependency Measures for Elderly People*. University of Sheffield: Joint Unit for Social Services Research/Community Care.

Wilkin, D., Hallam, L. and Doggett, M. (1992) *Measures of Need and Outcome for Primary Health Care*. Oxford: Oxford University Press.

Part IV

The roles and responsibilities of the researcher

Researching ageing in
different cultures

Margaret Boneham

Introduction

Recent trends in gerontological research suggest a growing awareness of the diverse nature of the older population. Differences between individuals with regard to class, gender and ethnicity are now acknowledged as being highly significant in accounting for variations in the experience of growing older. An understanding of ethnic diversity can enrich our appreciation of the process of growing older and help to provide a context for the study of important themes such as the impact of life transitions or changing intergenerational relations. Indeed, the value of such research is apparent when seen in the light of the ageing of the minority ethnic population in Britain combined with demands by minority communities and their older members for greater recognition. It could be argued that any book on researching ageing and later life would be incomplete without a chapter on the sociocultural context.

This important area is a controversial one as most key distinctions used to define the social identity of older people such as cultural, ethnic and racial are highly contested. There is an increase in consciousness and debates about such identities in British society and especially among minority communities. The emerging evidence points not to clear distinctive trends but 'the diversity, ambivalences and complexities that characterise the changing nature of ethnic identities' (Modood *et al.* 1994: 8).

Culture may be defined as 'a set of shared ideals, values and standards of behaviour' (Haviland 1996: 32). Research may focus on the explicit culture that is observed and understood by participants; also the implicit culture which is symbolic in nature. Culture is often falsely perceived as a static fixed product of tradition and this can result in a stereotyping of practices (Pfeffer 1998). Thus it is easy to present a fact file about the cultural characteristics of a community referring to the assumed religion, diet or dress of elders in the group when the actual degree of conformity to such practices varies according to gender, class and historical background. Different experiences of migration also illustrate this point. The contrasting experiences of a refugee as opposed to a well-established migrant or a recently arrived 'dependent' refugee will result in very different needs although all may be of the same age or cultural origin. Thus it is vital to recognize differences both within and between cultural groups. Indeed international migration in later life has important implications for the social care of older people (Blakemore 1999).

The attribution of social categories to older people is the result of the societal norms and context at any particular time. Distinctions of both race and ethnicity are socially constructed. The term *ethnicity* has its roots in pagan or heathen associations but has developed from this to encompass a subjective way of defining a sense of belonging to a group. There is a range of definitions but broad consensus that an ethnic identity comprises some if not all of the following four elements: a particular language; a sense of shared history and an association with a homeland (such as Sikh claims to Khalistan); a community link to a religion which may be special to the group or shared globally; and a distinctive culture (Blakemore and Boneham 1994). The importance of ethnicity is that it is contextual and open to change (Saifullah Khan 1982). This is relevant where ageing is concerned as ideas vary as to whether ethnic loyalties fade as older migrants adapt to their country of choice or, in contrast, increase in later life as a resource for coping with change in an unfamiliar world. The significance of ethnicity is vital in understanding the lives of black and Asian people, for instance, in making sense of the social life and expectations of old age; however, it is not a feature solely of minority ethnic groups. White majorities have ethnic preferences, e.g. those with Northern or Southern English, Welsh or Scottish backgrounds.

Ethnicity is sometimes used mistakenly as a synonym for race. However, whilst the two are linked they are not the same (Bhopal 1997). Race is a social construction which involves labels placed by outsiders on individuals. Racial judgements are based on making stereotypical assumptions about personal qualities. Race can be defined as 'a human group defined by itself or others as distinct by virtue of perceived common physical characteristics that are held to be inherent' (Cornell and Hartmann 1998: 24). The further stage, which develops from such definitions, is to assert that some racial groups are superior to others. This racism derives from a belief in inherent hierarchies and leads to negative discrimination, which dehumanizes and devalues individuals from a minority group who may be perceived as inferior. In using race, culture and ethnicity as explanations for differences in ageing it is important to reflect on the fact that such identities are the product of interactions which takes place between majority and minority groups. Research on ageing across cultures has to take account of the *power imbalance* in such interactions. Differential access to power between domin-ant and subordinate groups provides the context for the shaping of ageing studies. As Cornell and Hartmann (1998) argue, racism is more than pre-judice but is about conflicts over scarce resources. This applies patently in competition for jobs and housing. The experience of most older minority ethnic migrants is powerlessness; while applying for previous employment when jobs were restricted many were forced to accept low-status positions with poor pension entitlements. Thus research has focused on how poverty may further compound health disadvantage in old age for some older people from a minority culture (Boneham 2000).

Range of practice in this field

Reasons for neglect

In reviewing the range of practice in this field, it is clear that there has been a somewhat slow development of multicultural perspectives in geron-tology in the UK. The neglect in research is based on assumptions of low numbers, so that the issue is seen to be of minor concern and there is the perception of minority elders as being a small minority within a minority. Older people from minority ethnic groups have appeared to be 'invisible' and to look after their own. Until recently an under-utilization of health and welfare services was suspected but not proved (Blakemore and Boneham 1994). With respect to mental illness in older people the emphasis has been on whether depression or dementia actually exists in minority ethnic groups and how to measure the extent. Brownlie (1991) refers to the 'hidden problem' of dementia in minority ethnic groups in highlighting an apparently neglected area of research. Downs (2000), in contrast, recently stresses the growing interest which has emerged in gerontological studies in the sociocultural context of dementia and in discovering how dementia is in fact understood in non-Western societies.

Methodologies employed

Community surveys since the 1980s have helped to put minority ageing on the agenda and to present a gradually unfolding national picture of older people from minority cultures. Early surveys were modest in scope, of a small scale, initiated by local minority ethnic groups, rather than being on a government agenda. They were often funded using scant resources and were in the form of door-to-door interview surveys in urban areas, such as Birmingham (Bhalla and Blakemore 1981), London and Manchester (Barker 1984), Leicester (Donaldson 1986), Bristol (Fenton 1986) and London (Ebrahim *et al.* 1991).

Different methodologies employed in more recent studies have included analysis of quantitative data and more in-depth qualitative research. Some have used existing data sets to provide a national picture of minority groups and their socioeconomic position from which information on minority ageing could be derived. Modood and Berthoud (1997) utilized the Fourth National Survey to investigate the diversity of the material contexts of life in Britain for older minority ethnic people. Lowdell *et al.* (2000), in researching the health of minority ethnic elders in London, analysed Ethnicity Multiyear data from the General Household Survey as well as 1991 census returns. A recent project on the social exclusion of Chinese elders in London is an example of the use of semi-structured interviews where interviewees were asked to play an active role in defining their needs and formulating suggestions for meeting their problems (Wai Kam 2000). As part of the Better Government for Older People initiative (Better Government for Older People 1999) Sheffield University is undertaking a participatory and action research strategy using older women from different ethnic groups as researchers. They will also play a key role in publicizing the findings.

Work on Alzheimer's disease and ethnicity has focused on how to overcome the methodological difficulties in designing appropriate instruments for diagnosis. There are difficulties of translating emotions into English as, even with a translator, symptoms can be misinterpreted e.g. 'my heart is heavy' could indicate either a heart problem or depression. Rait and Burns (1998) have worked in Manchester on the assessment of instruments used in the diagnosis of depression and Alzheimer's disease. Lindesay's research in Leicester (1997) evaluated a Gujerati version of a tool to detect dementia with Gujerati speaking and British-born white older people. Marshall (1997) in Stirling, Scotland with the Dementia Study Group has maintained a database on Alzheimer's disease and ethnicity. Other current areas of research have focused on capturing the experiences of carers of minority ethnic dementia sufferers using in-depth interviews (Adamson 1999). The debate on cross-cultural issues in the measurement of dementia continues (Patel *et al.* 1998; Shah and Mukherjee 2000).

Sampling techniques

The population of minority elders in any given group is often unknown to service providers and can remain virtually invisible if the older members of the community neither access any services nor speak English. This remains a challenge for researchers regardless of ethnic background but especially

for those who may not share the same language as the older people themselves. Thus the methods used to identify a sample have been largely
convenience ones, through personal contact and community group leaders,
with some employing family practitioner lists and the electoral register.
Even in studies where the researcher is of the same ethnic group as the
older person, time has to be spent in gaining the confidence of local community members. For instance, in seeking possible participants for the
study of Chinese elders, access could only be achieved through gradually
establishing a rapport with members of the Chinese community and through
using the opportunity of existing social gatherings at McDonalds fast food
outlets to observe and interview participants (Wai Kam 2000).

Identifying a sample of older people from a minority community group is
especially important in assessing the health care needs of populations and
in planning health services. The whole issue of ethnic profiling in primary
care is debatable (Nazroo 1997) and there is no widespread systematic
recording of the ethnic origin of patients in order to inform decisions about
the purchasing of services. Examples of good practice do exist, such as the
development initiatives at Princes Park Health Centre, Liverpool (Lee *et al.*
2000), where participants have been assured that the results will be utilized
effectively to benefit minority community members.

Range of themes

Early studies provided information on how many older people existed and
what their welfare needs were. This demographic background indicated
in many cases high levels of unmet need for health and welfare services
coupled with a lack of knowledge of services. Many reports revealed family
breakdown, isolation, poverty, health disadvantage and lack of knowledge
of services. This was of value to local community groups in influencing
service providers in planning. However, there was a lack of acknowledgement of racism in the interaction between majority and minority groups;
the scale of the issues nationally was unknown; and arguably such studies
were not incorporating what the older people themselves really wanted to
say. More recently work has investigated the issue nationally, including
the role of racism in the provision of services and the participation of
older members of minority communities in defining their own agendas
(Torkington 1991; Eolas 1999; Joseph Rowntree Foundation 2001).

Case studies/examples

Two contrasting types of research with which the author was directly involved will illustrate methodological issues about gerontological work
in different cultures. The first is an individual piece of work for a PhD in

Leamington Spa involving in-depth work with a small number of elderly Sikh women over a period of five years. The second is a large-scale epidemiological study of prevalence rates for dementia and depression in a number of minority ethnic groups in inner city Liverpool for which the author acted as research assistant.

Case study 1: *The Leamington study*

Aims

The aim of the research was to investigate the impact of ageism and racism on the lives of twenty older Sikh women living in Leamington Spa, Warwickshire over a five-year period, especially focusing on the links with health and welfare agencies.

The process

The chosen methodology was action research and participant observation while the author was employed between 1982 and 1985 by the Manpower Services Commission as a community worker establishing a day centre for elderly Sikh women. Data collection involved mainly ethnographic techniques: fieldwork notes, detailed records of socioeconomic data and conversations with twenty women who attended the day centre and with whom there was twice-weekly contact. The major work to establish the centre by recruiting the older women and encouraging them to attend was completed by the Asian Punjabi-speaking support worker attached to the project. She acted as gatekeeper to the women, giving me access to their life histories, and I learned some Punjabi myself. The core of the data was thus a convenience sample of 20 case studies. There was also a reflective diary kept of all relevant events and membership of the Warwick District Community Relations Council, a special group at Social Services for the needs of ethnic minorities and the local Age Concern group. Some formal interviewing of older Asian men, statistical analysis of small area census data for the area and review of newspapers and committee minutes supplemented this over the research period.

Findings

The findings provided evidence to refute the common assumption that the extended Asian family universally supports its ageing members. Taking the 20 case studies as a whole, a quarter were not living in the extended family as a result of family tensions; 70 per cent spoke little English; 40 per cent were isolated as a result of living a considerable distance from the Temple and the remainder of the Sikh community, so being forced to spend long periods alone. An example follows:

Mrs Devi, aged 68, lived alone and spoke no English. She was over-weight, with diabetes, and had suffered a broken pelvis due to a road accident. Her husband had recently died and her son and daughter-in-law were in the process of migrating to Canada. Mrs Devi remained, unwilling to uproot herself again. Her daughter-in-law had come from Kenya to be married. She was an educated woman and was daunted by the task of being the sole carer of her mother-in-law. She felt guilty about leaving her elderly relative and only reluctantly accepted what she initially called 'interference' from social services. Home help was provided – the first Asian client in Leamington – but there were problems over Mrs Devi's expectations which were more in keeping with someone fulfilling a servant role. Mrs Devi frequently brought in financial issues for discussion at the day centre, such as large electricity bills and final rates demands. She had also been the object of racial harassment in the street in the form of verbal abuse and stone throwing.

There were a number of pressures which influenced the lives of the elderly Sikh women such as ageism, racism, restricted access to health and welfare services, internal ethnic divisions, class struggle and gender disparities (Boneham 1989). A model of multiple disadvantage which was developed confirmed and added to the double jeopardy theory of Dowd and Bengtson (1978). This had been derived in a USA context and had been confined largely to health and income.

In contrast the remainder of the case studies in Leamington demonstrated that real family support was available to the Sikh women and that a minority ethnic identity in fact enhanced the quality of life in old age. This is seen in the next example.

Mrs Singh was a frail but active 98-year-old living contentedly with her husband and extended family. Though bent and using a stick she could climb stairs unaided. Her granddaughter said she suffered from no major physical complaints. Her manner was alert and her movements vigorous. When visited at home she was surrounded by daughter-in-law, son, granddaughter and baby and they encouraged her to walk around the block frequently. She visited the day centre on a regular basis and enjoyed a party for her birthday there, being venerated as the oldest member.

Several of the women admitted that they had gained materially and in terms of security by migration compared with life in their native Punjab or in Africa in a situation of political instability. For seven out of the twenty cases the family offered regular and harmonious supportive contact. Where opportunities to meet were available, women of a common ethnic identity used each other as a resource, which enhanced the ageing process.

Thus there was some evidence which was contrary to the double jeopardy hypothesis, supporting instead the alternative 'age as leveller' theory (Kent 1971).

Practical lessons

The strength of the research was in the benefits resulting to the community itself and in particular derived by the older women themselves. A group was set up to meet twice weekly during the research process. This enabled the older Sikh women to relieve their social isolation and it still exists after fifteen years. Current organizers have just bid for lottery funding. The collaboration between the Asian support worker and myself ensured that the vital bridge with funding sources from the mainstream services was provided. In researching their needs it was possible to provide relevant data to social services, which supported the request for funding for transport to the day centre. The research was able to build up in-depth data about a hitherto 'invisible' group of people – notably women who spoke very little English. Their stories had not been told, and indeed it was assumed that their needs were already met within their extended families. As a result of their lack of English and different cultural practices older Asian women tended to be 'spoken for' rather than consulted about their views. The leaders of the Sikh community groups were male and the unique life histories of their female family members would not have been recorded otherwise. Their accounts provided further proof that Asian families do not universally care for their elders and that independent living is the desired preference for some – though not all.

One problem was the bias of the convenience sample – the women were self-selected by choosing to go to the centre. However, this was the only possible way of getting regular contact with a group of women. While ethnographic techniques lead to rich qualitative data, to complement this insight it is important to contextualize this sort of case study data with census findings and other documentary evidence.

Cross-cultural difficulties also arose which are found in any ethnographic work where the researcher is not of the same ethnic origin as the re-searched. There was an initial suspicion over a stranger taking notes in front of them due to fear of officialdom. However, these fears were soon allayed and care taken to record information at a different time. The need to engage in a range of mundane if pleasurable tasks such as making tea to gain credibility and an 'insider' perspective was also inherent in this type of research and has been documented elsewhere (Hammersley and Atkinson 1983).

Case study 2: *The Health and Ethnicity Project*

Aims

In contrast to the methodology employed in the previous research, the Health and Ethnicity Project was an epidemiological survey funded by Inner City Partnership for £90,000, which aimed to investigate the prevalence rates of depression and dementia in Liverpool's minority ethnic older people and their perceptions of mental health services across cultures. The main objective was to explore why so few persons aged 65 years and over from minority communities were in contact with psychogeriatric services in Liverpool. This is a city with a long-established record of immigration from the West Indies, Africa and the Far East, hence a black British population as well as thriving Chinese, West African and Somali communities. The issues to be addressed were whether older people from such communities existed at all; perhaps the minority populations had a more youthful age profile. Alternatively they might have been looked after by their extended family or community as some existing research suggests is common elsewhere (Kent 1971; Cool 1981). Other potential explanations for an underutilization were that they did not experience mental illness; they had not heard of mental health services or perceived them as inappropriate.

The process

To counteract the problems in achieving a complete enumeration the sample were identified using a combination of techniques; starting initially with the cooperation of GPs in areas of minority ethnic concentration in Liverpool 8. This had to be supplemented by lists of older people's luncheon clubs, 'snowballing' (asking a participant if they knew another) and a door knock exercise.

In order to measure the prevalence of depression and dementia a method was adopted which was similar to that used in a previous study in Liverpool: the ALPHA project. The core diagnostic instrument was the Geriatric Mental State Schedule, a semi-structured interview and computer diagnostic system covering a full range of psychiatric morbidity (Copeland *et al.* 1988). The MRC ALPHA study (Saunders *et al.* 1993) was a Medical Research Council-supported study of an age-stratified sample of 5222 older persons in Liverpool. The information obtained, it was hoped, would fill in a gap in existing ALPHA data where less than 1 per cent of interviews were conducted with minority ethnic groups. Members of various minority ethnic groups (Nigerian, Chinese, Somali, black British) were trained to interview, and matched with interviewee where possible. There was a two-phase design, first to screen, then consisting of an in-depth interview with those identified as 'cases' of depression and dementia, with their carers.

Findings

A total of 418 older people from the minority ethnic groups were interviewed, so the existence of a hitherto under-researched group was proved.
The sample consisted of 55 per cent men aged 65–74 years old, 22 per cent
men of 75 years and over, 16 per cent of women aged 65–74 and 7 per
cent women aged 75 years and older. This is a far higher percentage of
men than in the older population of Liverpool as a whole and reflects the
high numbers of seamen and Chinese restaurateurs who have settled in
Liverpool. The prevalence rates for all different ethnic groups for depression and dementia were as high as for white elders in the city, showing the
extent of underutilization of current psychogeriatric services and considerable unmet need. The reasons why sufferers were not coming forward
were that GPs were not referring them on and that services were perceived
as culturally inappropriate. Further details are to be found in publications
such as Boneham *et al.* (1994, 1997) and McCracken *et al.* (1997).

Practical lessons

A number of interesting lessons regarding recruitment of participants and
survey design can be derived from the experience of this research. First,
with regard to the use of lists of names, it was possible to use general
practice information from age/sex registers but in the absence of a national
ethnic monitoring system this had to be done with the cooperation of GP
practices where individuals could be involved in identifying their own
ethnicity. In general, regardless of source, names from lists are insufficient
to identify ethnicity – Punjabi or Hindu names are distinctive but impossible for those older people with a black British identity. A name can be
misleading if a woman has married someone from a minority ethnic
background. Furthermore, lists may soon become obsolete. Of the names
obtained through the general practice lists, 40 per cent could not be traced
mainly because the addresses did not exist. This inaccuracy has been noticed
in other studies in inner city areas because of the amount of migration due
to demolition of housing and redevelopment schemes (Smith 1989).

   Another lesson to be remembered for research with minority elders in
inner city areas is the problem of identifying the sample and the need to
anticipate persistence, necessitating going beyond obvious gatekeepers.
24 per cent of the sample interviewed had to be obtained from other
sources such as door knocking and snowballing, i.e. through a combination
of methods. A large degree of detective work and time was involved in
consulting and getting to know different communities in order to obtain
a sample. This was only possible with the cooperation of key community
figures.

   In terms of epidemiological difficulties, the type of interview schedule
used may be problematic. This study indicated that there might have been
an overestimate in the prevalence of dementia in those not speaking the

dominant language. Elevated levels of dementia in Chinese elders could have been an artefact of the diagnostic instrument used, in this case the Geriatric Mental State Schedule. There is a need for the further development of validated assessment instruments for screening depression and dementia in specific minority ethnic communities because the existing ones are based on a European model, as Rait *et al.* argue (1996).

Another area of concern was in the design of the initial project. There was some criticism by members of minority groups in the statutory services that they had not been involved in the original design. They viewed research of this kind across cultures as having the danger of further stigmatizing and fuelling racial prejudice. They argued that media reporting of high levels of mental illness in older people from minority groups might have highlighted ethnicity as a 'problem'. It is especially important that power relations between majority and minority cultures are acknowledged and that disenfranchized groups see tangible benefits where possible in the policy implications of the findings. Consultation has to begin at the design stage and be continued through an appropriate advisory group with a process of continually negotiating access, checking the understanding throughout of both the researchers and the participants. The term 'research project' may have negative associations in areas regularly the object of scrutiny such as Liverpool 8 (Lee *et al.* 2000). The objectives of research based at health centres in such areas has to be explicitly to enable an evaluation of service provision, with patients, the community and the Primary Health Care team having joint ownership.

Further work of interest on ageing and ethnicity

Action research of the type described earlier is best for students in social care or institutional settings such as hospitals and day centres seeking to discover more about local needs. Gathering such data about minority ethnic communities is essential evidence to enable Primary Care Trusts to address inequalities and purchase suitable provision for older people. Indeed, the National Service Framework for Older People stresses the importance of research to understand the needs of older people from black and minority ethnic communities (Department of Health 2001), especially with regard to developing more accessible and appropriate mental health services. It is essential to work not merely from existing academic literature about the assumed particular culture as this may suggest an apparent homogeneity, which does not exist. Researchers working across cultures have been in danger of perpetuating stereotypes, ignoring internal differences and contributing to the 'othering' of minority group members (Modood *et al.* 1994). Information concerning cultural practices may be out of date, under-represent women or refer more to traditional religious practice rather than the real lived existence of people. The way to gain understanding is to build close and meaningful links with the community, first to establish whether it is a real community or a diverse number of communities and then gradually to seek to understand how ageing is played out in a unique cultural context.

The ethnicity of the researcher is an issue here. The necessity to match interviews by gender and culture is an interesting point of debate. Does one have to be a member of the cultural group to research it? It is possible for an 'outsider' to gather valid data successfully by making strong contacts with stakeholders such as community and religious leaders and devoting time to building up confidence and trust with them and other relevant persons. However, most leaders are male and may be used to speaking on behalf of their female family members, especially if they are non-English speakers. It is especially appropriate for research on gender and minority ageing to closely involve women who share the cultural background of the group under study to ensure that they set the agenda, elicit women's views and experiences directly and use the results appropriately.

Conclusion

The cultural context for ageing adds an important dimension to geronto-logical research. Where minority older people are not in contact with existing service providers there may be challenges for any researcher in obtaining a representative sample and in gaining credibility for his or her research. A diversity of approaches is necessary, working with community groups and key workers in order to recruit respondents, especially in inner city areas. Some degree of matching of ethnicity and gender in interviewing is important, especially with non-English speaking women. Minority communities have suffered in the past from having their needs dismissed through ignorance or apathy and not being involved in the design of research about their own members. The full participation of elders of minority ethnic communities should be the model in research and policy making, leading to the better and more appropriate purchasing of services by Primary Care Trusts.

References

Adamson, J. (1999) Carers and dementia among African/Caribbean and South Asian families, *Generations Review*, 9 (3):12–14.

Barker, J. (1984) *Black and Asian Old People in Britain*. Mitcham: Age Concern.

Better Government for Older People (1999) *Making it Happen: Report of the First Year of the Better Government for Older People Programme 1998–1999*. Wolverhampton: Better Government for Older People.

Bhalla, A. and Blakemore, K. (1981) *Elders of Minority Ethnic Groups*. Birmingham: AFFOR.

Bhopal, R. (1997) Is research into ethnicity and health racist, unsound or important science?, *British Medical Journal*, 314: 1751–5.

Blakemore, K. (1999) International migration in later life: social care and policy implications, *Ageing and Society*, 19: 761–74.

Blakemore, K. and Boneham, M. (1994) *Age, Race and Ethnicity*. Buckingham: Open University Press.

Boneham, M. (1989) Ageing and ethnicity in Britain: the case of elderly Sikh women in a Midlands town, *New Community*, 15(3): 447–59.

Boneham, M. (2000) Shortchanging black and minority ethnic elders, in J. Bradshaw and R. Sainsbury (eds) *Experiencing Poverty*. Aldershot: Ashgate.

Boneham, M., Saunders, P., Copeland, J. *et al.* (1994) Age, race and mental health: Liverpool's elderly people from ethnic minorities, *Health and Social Care in the Community*, 2: 113–16.

Boneham, M., Williams, K., Copeland, J. *et al.* (1997) Elderly people from ethnic minorities in Liverpool: mental illness, unmet need and barriers to service use, *Health and Social Care in the Community*, 5(3): 173–80.

Brownlie, J. (1991) *A Hidden Problem? Dementia amongst Minority Ethnic Groups*. University of Stirling: Dementia Services.

Cool, L. (1981) Ethnicity and aging – continuity through change in elderly Corsicans, in C. Fry (ed.), *Community Planning for an Aging Society*. New York, NY: Hutchinson and Ross.

Copeland, J. (1988) Quantifying clinical observation – geriatric mental state (AGECAT package), in J. Wattis and I. Hindmarch (eds) *Psychological Assessments of the Elderly*. Edinburgh: Churchill Livingstone.

Cornell, S. and Hartmann, D. (1998) *Ethnicity and Race*. London: Pine Forge Press.

Department of Health (2001) *National Service Framework for Older People*. London: Department of Health.

Donaldson, L.J. (1986) Health and social status of elderly Asians: a community survey, *British Medical Journal*, 293: 1079–84.

Dowd, J. and Bengtson, V. (1978) Ageing in minority populations: an examination of the double jeopardy hypothesis, *Journal of Gerontology*, 33(3): 427–36.

Downs, M. (2000) Dementia in a socio cultural context: an idea whose time has come, *Ageing and Society*, 20: 369–75.

Ebrahim, S., Patel, N. and Coats, M. (1991) Prevalence and severity of morbidity among Gujerati Asian elders: a controlled comparison, *Family Practitioner* 8(1): 57–62.

Eolas (1999) *Health and Social Care for Older Black and Minority Ethnic Residents of Sefton*. Liverpool: Personal Social Services.

Fenton, S. (1986) *Race, Health and Welfare: Afro Caribbean South Asian People in Central Bristol*. Bristol: Dept of Sociology, University of Bristol.

Fernando, S. (1988) *Race and Culture in Psychiatry*. London: Croom Helm.

Hammersley, M. and Atkinson, P. (1983) *Ethnography: Principles in Practice*. London: Tavistock.

Haviland, W. (1996) *Social Anthropology*. New York, NY: Harcourt Brace.

Joseph Rowntree Foundation (2001) http://www.jrf.org.uk/funding/priorities/scdc.asp (accessed 27 June 2002).

Kent, D. (1971) The elderly in minority groups: variant patterns of ageing, *The Gerontologist*, 11(1): 26–9.

Lee, B., Gardner, K., Jones, B. *et al.* (eds) (2000) *Ethnicity Profiling in Primary Care: A Princes Park Model.* Liverpool: Public Health Sector, Liverpool John Moores University.

Lindesay, J., Jagger, C., Hibbett, M.J., Peet, S.M. and Moledina, S.F. (1997) Knowledge, uptake and availability of health and social services among Asian Gujerati and white elderly persons, *Ethnicity and Health*, 1: 56–69.

Lowdell, C., Evandrou, M. *et al.* (2000) *Health of Ethnic Minority Elders in London.* London: Health of Londoners Project.

McCracken, C., Boneham, M., Copeland, C. *et al.* (1997) Prevalence of dementia and depression among elderly people in black and ethnic minorities, *British Journal of Psychiatry*, 171: 269–73.

Marshall, M. (1997) Introduction, in M. Marshall (ed.) *State of the Art in Dementia Care.* London: Centre for Policy on Ageing.

Modood, T. and Berthoud, R. (1997) *Ethnicity in Britain: Diversity and Disadvantage.* London: Policy Studies Institute.

Modood, T., Beishon, S. and Virdee, S. (1994) *Changing Ethnic Identities.* London: Policy Studies Institute.

Nazroo, J.Y. (1997) *The Health of Britain's Ethnic Minorities.* London: Policy Studies Institute.

Patel, N., Mirza, N., Lindblad, P., Amstrup, K. and Samaoli, O. (1998) *Dementia and Minority Ethnic Older People.* Leeds: Russell House Publishing.

Pfeffer, N. (1998) Theories of race, ethnicity and culture, *British Medical Journal*, 317: 1381–4.

Rait, G. and Burns, A. (1998) A screening for depression and cognitive impairment in older people from ethnic minorities, *Age and Ageing*, 27: 271–5.

Rait, G., Burns, A. and Chew, C. (1996) Age, ethnicity and mental illness: a triple whammy, *British Medical Journal*, 313: 1347.

Saifullah Khan, V.S. (1982) The role of the culture of dominance in structuring the experience of ethnic minorities, in C. Husband (ed.) *Race in Britain.* London: Hutchinson.

Saunders, P., Copeland, J., Dewey, M. *et al.* (1993) The prevalence of dementia, depression and the neuroses in an elderly community sample: findings from the Liverpool MRC Alpha Study, *International Journal of Epidemiology*, 22: 838–47.

Shah, A. and Mukherjee, S. (2000) Cross cultural issues in the measurement of behavioural and psychological signs and symptoms of dementia, *Aging and Mental Health*, 4(3): 244–52.

Smith, A. (1989) The politics of inadequate registers, *British Medical Journal*, 299: 458.

Torkington, N. (1991) *Black Health: A Political Issue.* Liverpool: Catholic Association for Racial Justice.

Wai Kam, Y. (2000) *Chinese Older People: A Need for Social Inclusion in Two Communities.* Bristol: The Policy Press/Joseph Rowntree Foundation.

13

Ethical issues in researching later life

Mary Gilhooly

Introduction

In one sense there is nothing special about researching later life, or research with older people. Most older people live independent lives, are self-
determining, and are competent to decide whether or not to take part in
research. Thus, they should be treated in the same way that one would
treat any other adult asked to take part in research, and the ethical issues
that arise are no different when conducting research with older people
than they are when conducting research with younger adults (Kapp and
Bigot 1985). However, as we age we are more likely to suffer from a variety
of impairments, physical and mental, which might affect our *competence* to
consent to research. In addition, in advanced old age many people find
they can no longer live independently in the community and must, therefore, move into residential or nursing home care. These environments pose
special ethical issues in relation to *voluntariness*, a second component of valid
consent for participation in research. Finally, advanced age may create
special problems in relation to the giving and understanding of *information*,
the third aspect of valid consent (Ratzan 1980).

Valid consent is essential to the ethical practice of social science research.
Unlike animal research, there is no legislation covering research with
humans. This is because, unlike animals, competent adults are assumed to
be free to refuse to take part in research which they perceive as risky or of
no benefit. However, because there is an inherent conflict between the need
to conduct research and the need to protect people from possible harm,

research ethics committees now scrutinize research conducted by staff in universities, hospital trusts, and health boards/authorities. The scrutiny of research proposals should take into consideration four main ethical principles and a set of derivative principles, give prominence to the elements of valid consent, and review study design to ensure that the proposed study is of sufficient scientific merit to justify subjecting study participants to possible physical and psychological risks.

Ethical principles

Four principles are relevant to the practice of ethical research:

1 Non-maleficence – do no harm;
2 Beneficence – do positive good;
3 Justice – treat people fairly; and
4 Autonomy – have respect for people.

There are also a number of derivative moral rules, namely fidelity, veracity, confidentiality and privacy. It is worth considering the application of these four principles to the research setting and noting some of the expectations which are currently held about the ways in which research should be conducted.

Guiding ethical principles

Non-maleficence

Beneficence

Justice

Autonomy

Non-maleficence – do no harm

Clearly some procedures which are undertaken for research purposes can cause discomfort or a degree of 'harm' to the research subject. This is as true of psychological harm which might result from questionnaires, and interviews which contain embarrassing or sensitive questions, as it is of more invasive procedures such as blood sampling. It is clear that the amount of discomfort or 'harm' and its likely impact should, therefore, be a key consideration in the ethical scrutiny of research. Research which carries a risk of distress should only be conducted by investigators with training in managing distressed study participants. Particular care should be exercised in decisions about what types of research can be conducted by undergraduate students.

Where potential psychological harm is involved it is important to provide some means of addressing this after the research procedure has been undertaken, or in some cases after the research study as a whole has been completed. In the conduct of such research, therefore, the researcher is obliged to plan for the following where appropriate: the provision of counselling if the research subject is likely to become distressed by the topic (an example might include elderly people invited to discuss issues such as death and dying) and advice about services or help which the participant might solicit as a result of discussing needs which are not being met.

Beneficence – do positive good

Social science research rarely offers direct benefit for the participant. However, social science research should be of potential scientific or practical value. That is, it must address an important question and be feasible and well designed.

Autonomy – show respect for the right to self-determination

The principle of autonomy is regarded by many as the most important principle in research ethics. Respect for autonomy implies respect for the potential participant's right to self-determination. Self-determination is the shaping of one's self by one's choices. Although many philosophers argue that no one is totally self-determining, it is also argued that self-determination is part of the subjective reality of life, and that few things mean more to us than this freedom.

Justice – treat people fairly

Treating people fairly means treating everyone equally. It means that the researcher is obliged to offer the same explanations and same treatment to all research subjects irrespective of their status. It might, for example, be tempting to assume that a class of schoolchildren could be asked to fill in a questionnaire without offering them the same explanations or freedom not to participate as a group of adults. Justice also requires that classes or groups of people are not exploited for research purposes. This includes people living in institutions. The case for justice is not quite the same as voluntariness in consent. It would be unfair if certain groups were used repeatedly for research just because they were convenient.

Valid consent

The law, professional research guidelines, and research ethics committees require that people consent to take part in research. For consent to be valid it must be informed, voluntary and competent (Kennedy 1988). It is through informed and voluntary consent that individuals exercise self-determination in relation to research participation. Because respect for autonomy is regarded as of prime importance, awareness and understanding of the three main elements of consent is central to ethical research.

Informed consent

The term 'informed consent' stems from a legal doctrine in the United States that consent to treatment will only be valid if patients have been given the information that they need to make an autonomous decision. The US legal standard is that of what the ordinary person would want or need to give consent (*Canterbury v. Spence*). In the United Kingdom the 'professional standard' holds (*Sidaway v. Board of Governers of the Bethlem Royal and the Maudsley Hospital*). This means that professionals need only give the type and amount of information that others would normally give (Brazier 1987; McLean 1989).

Although the requirement for information disclosure for consent in the UK seems rather less respectful of autonomy than that in the United States, it must be kept in mind that the standard for consent to research participation is higher than that for treatment. It is accepted that in research there are very few exceptions to the requirement that research participants should be fully informed. Any exceptions to this requirement must be justified.

In bio-medicine potential study participants must be informed of both the risks and the benefits of study participation. Interestingly, it is relatively rare for social researchers to consider, let alone inform participants about, the risks and benefits of participation. Because social research rarely involves physical risks researchers often do not think about risks. Perhaps because social research rarely involves direct benefits to participants, social researchers also do not contemplate discussion of the benefits of study participation. Over the past twenty years participation rates in social research have declined dramatically. Perhaps if we were better at marketing the benefits of participation in such research we could improve response rates. Interestingly, we have found that it is often the case that older people are more, rather than less, likely to agree to take part in studies by young postgraduate students, than those where more mature research assistants collect the data. Older people often comment that they will participate to 'help' the young student with his or her studies. Presumably providing this type of help to young people is viewed as beneficial to the older person.

Information leaflets

Providing information to potential research participants is more difficult and complex than might be supposed. In medical research potential research participants must be given Patient Information Sheets outlining the aims and procedures and risks and benefits, if any. However, there are no national guidelines as to exactly what must go in an Information Sheet, nor is there guidance for researchers on how to write an Information Sheet. Some Health Boards and Trusts have a set protocol for Patient Information Sheets. In the past patients were often given an information sheet to read which was attached to the Consent Form; it was then taken away when the consent form was signed. Nowadays it is expected that the information sheet will be a separate document which can be retained by the study participant.

There are no fixed rules about the level and nature of information that must be provided to potential participants in social gerontology research. Many years of research in social gerontology have, however, led me to the view that the best way to provide information is in a three-fold leaflet, using a question and answer format. The questions that we ask and answer are listed in Box 13.1. It is important that the leaflet gives names, addresses and telephone numbers of members of the research team who can be contacted.

Box 13.1   Information leaflet questions

- What is the purpose of this research?
- Who is doing the research?
- What do I have to do?
- Why choose me?
- Is the information confidential?
- Can I refuse to answer questions?

There are other questions that might need answering, depending on the nature of the study. For example,

- Can someone be with me during the interview?
- How are the interviews arranged?
- Who do I contact for further information before I make up my mind?

Sometimes we include photographs of the research worker if the study involves home interviews. 'Stranger Danger' campaigns by the police mean that older people are most reluctant to let people they do not know into their homes; photographs on information leaflets are therefore reassuring for older people.

Testing of the information leaflets is very important. Researchers need to ensure that potential study participants find the leaflet attractive, acceptable and understandable. Researchers may have to rewrite and retest the information leaflet several times.

Understanding

It is one thing to give potential research participants information; it is another to ensure that they understand that information. Should the information given be that which most people would understand, or what each individual participant can understand? While it might be relatively easy to give information verbally at a level which could be understood by most individuals, it is harder to ensure that information is understandable to particular individuals when it is in a written form. Good research practice requires that information is given both verbally and in a written form whenever possible.

There are a number of common-sense methods of ensuring that written information is understandable to 'most' potential participants. First, it should be jargon-free. Second, information leaflets should be tested for 'reading ease'. Recent word-processing packages include different methods of testing for reading ease. Reading ease formulae will tell you what proportion of the population will be able to understand the text as well as the reading level required for understanding. Third, the information to be given to potential participants should be rigorously tested in pilot studies; pilot study participants should be asked how understandable the information is and how it could be improved. Potential participants should, of course, be given an opportunity to ask questions about the research before agreeing to take part.

Voluntary consent

For consent to research participation to be valid, consent must be voluntary. Conceptualizing and defining voluntariness is more difficult than most researchers realize. This is also the aspect of consent which is often most practically problematic and where researchers are most likely to display behaviours which may border on the unethical. Researchers tend to view their research as extremely important and, hence, find it difficult to accept that their attempts to obtain compliance might not be ethically justified.

The Belmont Report (1978) distinguishes between coercion, undue influence and unjustifiable pressures as follows. *Coercion* occurs when an overt threat of harm is intentionally presented by one person to another in order to obtain compliance. *Undue influence*, by contrast, occurs through an offer of an excessive, unwarranted, inappropriate or improper reward or other overture in order to obtain compliance. *Unjustifiable pressure* usually occurs when persons in position of authority or commanding influence – especially where possible sanctions are involved – urge a course of action for a participant.

Where does unjustifiable persuasion end and undue influence begin? What counts as undue influence? Examples of undue influence include actions such as manipulating a person's choice through the controlling influence of a close relative. A variety of 'pressures' can also affect decision making: examples include wishing to please a doctor, social workers or other professional who has helped or might help the person; too little time for reflection; payment of fees and expenses; and possibly even features of participant's mental state (e.g. participants may agree to participate in research which is unpleasant or hazardous because they think they are unworthy and should be punished). Features of the environment may also affect the voluntary nature of consent. Older people in residential or nursing home care may be bored and welcome a chance to speak with another person – any person and on any topic.

There are a number of practical ways of ensuring that participants do not feel pressured or coerced into taking part in research. First, potential participants must be told that services will not be denied to them if they do not take part, nor will refusal to participate result in any other form of discrimination. Second, researchers must also be aware that their status alone may put pressure on people to participate in research. Acknowledgement of this has led to a policy in many medical schools where medical students are not allowed to take part in medical research. This is because medical students may find it difficult to say no when asked by professors, lecturers or clinicians to take part in research. Even students new to university might find it difficult to say no if a more senior student or member of staff asks them to take part in research.

Because many research projects might involve some element of pressure, it is becoming more common to require that participants, especially patients, 'opt in' to studies. For example, a general practitioner might write to patients asking if they would be willing to take part in a named researcher's study, and asking them to return a postcard indicating willingness to participate, with non-returns regarded as refusals. Such procedures have been adopted because of increasing awareness of the difficulty people have in saying 'no'. In other words, ethical practice requires that the researcher make it easy for people to refuse to participate. Of course, making it easy to refuse has been found to lead to low response rates which has been damaging to research.

Giving potential research participants time to consider whether or not they want to take part in the research is now regarded as important in ensuring that consent is voluntary. In the same way that many surgeons now give patients who are offered risky treatments the opportunity to make decisions at home, rather than in the hospital where the mere presence of doctors and nurses might be coercive, social science researchers should think carefully about methods that ensure that consent is voluntary. This is especially important in any research that might distress study participants.

Research participants must also be assured that consent can be revoked at any time. Although it is common practice to tell people at the beginning of a study that they can refuse to answer questions, or that they can terminate an interview at any time, one suspects that it is rare for an interviewer, for example, to reconfirm that the participant wishes to continue, or at the end of an interview to ask study participants for permission to take audio tapes and interview schedules away.

Research in nursing homes and residential care

People who reside in institutions (e.g. old people in nursing homes) are also under pressure to participate in research. The boredom that many people experience in institutions may be part of a subtle pressure for research participation. Recognition of the pressures on prisoners to take part in research in the United States, led to an almost blanket ban on research in prisons. However, more recently prisoners in the United States have argued that the ban on research participation is discriminatory. Prisoners' organizations have argued that research participation gives prisoners an opportunity to feel that they are helping to contribute something to the greater good of society. Although it might seem odd to mention this issue in a book on social gerontology, there is a growing population of older people in prisons and recent years have seen a developing interest in the nature of social ageing in unusual environments such as prisons.

Competent consent

Potential research participants need to be competent (or 'capax' as we say in Scotland) to consent before consent can be regarded as valid. Competence is not 'all-or-nothing'. Someone with a learning disability would be regarded as competent to decide what to eat in a restaurant, but his or her competence to consent to marriage might be questioned. A person with moderate dementia might be regarded as competent to answer simple questions about the quality of food in a day hospital, but not competent to consent to take part in a randomized controlled drug trial. Thus, competence is *task specific* (Beauchamp 1991). Because competence is task-specific, it is impossible to specify universal criteria for tests of competence. This means that researchers must think carefully about the criteria for competence to consent to participation in their particular study.

An interesting issue in health services research, as well as social research, is whether or not any physically ill older person is capable of consenting to take part in research. Pain, the effects of medications, nausea and other symptoms of physical illness are all likely to impact on decision making. The social deprivation that older people in residential care, nursing homes, or long-stay hospital wards experience may affect capacity to consent to research. Although it is sometimes suggested that ageist attitudes lead younger people to assume that older people experience diminished memories, thinking and problem-solving skills, pressure on researchers to obtain study participants makes it highly likely that competence will be assumed. Sometimes it is so difficult to obtain study participants that researchers ignore signs that study participants may not have had the capacity to give valid consent.

Justifying non-consensual research

Research with people with Alzheimer's disease, or one of the many other disorders that diminish cognitive functioning in old age, raises special legal, ethical and methodological issues (Dubler 1985; Dworkin 1987). As noted above, valid consent requires that the study participant be competent to consent. Unless certain legal mechanisms are put in place, adult children or other adults (e.g. managers of nursing homes) cannot give consent for people with diminished capacity to take part in research. While it is good practice to ask relatives for consent, without the appropriate legal mechanisms in place such consent has no legal standing. Does this mean, therefore, that no research, medical or social, can be done with older people with diminished capacity? Some would argue that the answer is yes. Others would argue that research on non-consenting older people can proceed provided it can be ethically justified.

A number of arguments have been put forward to justify conducting research on non-consenting people with dementia. First, it could be argued that the incidence of dementia has reached epidemic proportions and that research to find either a cure or a means of 'control' is needed in order to prevent the dementing from becoming a threat to the delivery of medical, educational and social services to other groups of disabled persons or to younger members of society. Second, it could be argued that dementia is such a degrading disorder for the sufferer, and is so feared by elderly people that, were they able to consent to research, the elderly would gladly do so in order to prevent others suffering in a similar way.

Another argument that aims to justify research with older people who are not competent to consent stems from utilitarianism, an ethical theory that puts forward the case for judging the rightness and wrongness of an action according to its consequences. Thus, an action is right if it leads to the 'greatest good for the greatest number'. The argument for including non-consenting in research, an act which would under most circumstances not be regarded as ethical, would be justified on the grounds that the knowledge gained would be beneficial for future generations of older people and, hence, would lead to welfare maximization. The fundamental premise is that, because we have all benefited from medical research, we all have a duty to help future generations by participating in research (Rights and Legal Protection Sub-Committee, Scottish Action on Dementia 1992).

Assuming that research with non-consenting older people can be morally justified, it is, however, important that an attempt is made to obtain some form of consent from the older person with cognitive impairment. At the very least, research should not proceed if the potential participant objects, protests, or in some way exhibits distress.

Consent forms

Consent forms are required in health settings for most research projects. Hospital or health board research ethics committees often have standard forms which researchers are required to use. Consent forms have no legal standing. While they may provide the researcher with some 'evidence' that the participant had consented to take part in the research, the participant might be able to demonstrate that consent was, nevertheless, invalid because he or she had been coerced into taking part in the research or had not understood the information given.

The practice of using consent forms in social science research has increased in the last decade although there is still disagreement as to how far this practice should be extended. For example, should people taking part in interviews be required to sign a consent form? Although it might seem a useful 'safeguard' to have an interviewee sign a consent form, asking participants to sign such forms often raises suspicions about the nature of the research. This may reduce the likelihood that people will agree to take part in research. It is my view that most social science research does not require the use of written consent forms. Studies involving patients need to follow the advice of the hospital trust or health board/authority research ethics committee as to whether or not written consent is required.

Confidentiality and privacy

Confidentiality is important for three reasons (Harris 1985). First, there is an implied, and indeed often real, 'contract' between the study participant and the researcher. The research participant gives information on the understanding that it will not be divulged to others. Second, there is a strong utilitarian argument for keeping the confidences of study participants. If the research community did not keep confidences, in no time we would find that people would be unwilling to take part in our research. Rights of privacy also imply a duty of non-disclosure. A right to privacy includes personal control over information about oneself and over access to that information. Without such control trust in the research community would diminish.

Researchers routinely tell potential participants that data will be treated as highly confidential, and that data stored on a computer will be anonymized. To study participants, confidentiality tends to mean that only the interviewer will access the audio tapes, transcripts and data. This is rarely the case as most research now involves a team of grant holders and often more than one research assistant. Increasingly data are also archived by funding bodies (for example the ESRC) and can be made accessible to other researchers at a later date. Quantitative data can easily be anonymized, but qualitative data (audio tapes and transcripts, quotes, etc.) are much harder to anonymize.

It is also worth noting that confidentiality and anonymity are not the same. As the Chair of a Research Ethics Committee I often find myself having to tell researchers that a postal questionnaire which is numbered, and where the number is attached to a name, is not an anonymous questionnaire. To be truly anonymous the researchers must have no way of identifying the respondent. If researchers choose to number questionnaires in order to follow up non-responders, they must not describe the survey as anonymous. At best the survey can only be described as confidential.

A great deal of the research conducted by social gerontologists involves sensitive issues. Even when not asked, the intimate nature of interviews often means that study participants reveal information that they are not directly asked about. While some participants might regard the interview as somewhat therapeutic, many come to regret telling interviewers about details of their lives and families. In one of my recent projects a study participant asked to have the tapes and interview schedule returned to her so that they could be destroyed. The interview had been conducted on a Friday and she had worried all weekend about personal and family details that she had revealed. When she arrived on Monday to collect the tape and interview schedule she was clearly very distressed. We were somewhat mystified by this incident because the study did not, in our view, enquire into particularly private matters and the participant had not revealed information that we viewed as especially personal. Nevertheless, this incident raised our awareness of the need to tell study participants not only that information would be confidential and that they were free not to answer questions, but also that the data and tapes would be returned or destroyed if they changed their minds at some later date.

Informing study participants that material gathered during interviews can be returned does, of course, create difficulties for research managers. The material most likely to be requested for return is that which is most difficult to obtain. It is demoralizing for research assistants to expend effort and time obtaining study participants, conducting in-depth and potentially stressful interviews, and then to have to give back or destroy the data. More importantly, suggesting that materials can be returned might suggest to potential study participants that their privacy will be severely invaded, even when the nature of the study demands little in the way of self-revelation. In the same way that asking people to sign consent forms to participate in interviews has the potential for reducing response rates, telling participants that they can ask for the data to be returned or destroyed may also reduce response rates. There are no easy solutions to these more complex managerial problems.

During confidential interviews one may also obtain information which may lead to conflicts between the duty to respect confidentiality and other duties. For example, one might learn of the abuse of an elderly dementing relative from a caregiver, or even perhaps of other more serious criminal activities. Obligations to minimize suffering and injury to others is a legitimate reason for breaching confidentiality, but the researcher must think very carefully about the consequences of breaking a confidence. An elderly woman might be aware that her caregiving daughter-in-law is stealing her money and might be deeply unhappy about episodes of verbal abuse, but might prefer the loss of money and verbal abuse to having to move into institutional care.

Controlling and monitoring research

As noted at the start of this chapter, there is an inherent conflict in research which is conducted by health and social care professionals, and indeed by academic researchers. Research is needed in order to improve treatments and interventions and to gain a greater understanding of the position of older people in society, an understanding which will lead to an improved quality of life in old age. In addition, to further their careers, academics and health and social care professionals increasingly need to do research (Downie and Calman 1987). One can expect the pressure to do research to increase. Thus, researchers may not be the best people to judge whether or not their own research is ethical. Control and scrutiny by those outside the researchers' own profession, as well as the lay public, is necessary to ensure that the research participant's rights are protected (Makarushka and McDonald 1979; Waters 1980).

Research ethics committees

The first port of call for researchers should be their university ethics committee or the research ethics committee of their employer (health board/

authority, hospital trust, social work department). Many universities now produce guidelines, as well as recommend other sources of information on the principles of ethical research. The distinctions between these three types of activities noted above – research, audit and practice-orientated activity – is important because audit and practice-oriented activity frequently do not require ethical committee approval. However, it is important that researchers consult their employers' guidelines to ensure that they seek ethics committee approval where this is required.

Although research ethical committees perform a useful monitoring service, the various committees view their role mainly as one of protecting people from exploitation and concentrate on the 'ethics' of consent and issue of coercion. Other committees see their role more as scrutinizing the research protocol for scientific merit. While it is true that research which is badly designed and, hence, unlikely to reveal anything of merit is de facto 'unethical', committees which focus primarily on design may fail to note elements of the procedure which are unethical on other grounds. Research on the activities of ethics committees has found considerable variation in how they operate, the nature of their enquiries, the forms used, and the expertise and discipline base of the ethics committees (Thompson *et al.* 1981; Gilbert *et al.* 1989; Neuberger 1992).

Guidelines

Professional bodies such as the British Psychological Society, the British Sociological Association, and the Medical Research Council all produce guidelines on the ethics of research and it is wise for researchers to examine the ethical guidelines produced by their professional bodies. Increasingly general textbooks also have chapters on research ethics which are a useful starting point for those new to research in social gerontology. Universities and hospital trusts may also have written guidelines on the principles of ethical research.

Although valuable as a clear statement of the aims and limitations which should be borne in mind by all those involved in research, ethical guidelines are of little use as a direct method of control over the behaviour of researchers (McLean and Maher 1983). Ethical guidelines are backed by few legal sanctions in the event of a breach of a code. While it might be the case that a very serious breach of ethical guidelines might lead to dismissal of a researcher, it is unlikely that a university or hospital trust would dismiss a member of staff who conducted a relatively risk-free study (e.g. a survey) without having obtained ethical committee approval. Moreover, unless there is an explicit policy on sanctions for breach of guidelines, employers would find that there was little that they could do in the event of research proceeding without ethical approval.

The duties of researchers

Another way of looking at the ethics of research is to note researchers' duties. The duties of researchers are:

- to ensure that consent is informed;
- to ensure that participation is voluntary and in no way coerced, and that withdrawal is allowed at any time;
- to ensure confidentiality; and
- to ensure that the benefits of the study to the participant or society outweigh the risks to the participant.

Grant holders and supervisors must also ensure that research assistants and students are aware of the ethical principles that guide research and that, where research might cause distress, staff are adequately trained to deal with distress.

Although research ethics committees have the power to give ethical approval, and will to some extent monitor research projects via interim reports, much depends on the commitment of researchers to conduct ethical research. Researchers are often under considerable pressure from funding councils to ensure high response rates, pressures which can easily cause researchers to show less than ideal respect for voluntary consent or even competent consent. There may also be a tendency to slip into giving evasive answers to questions in order to persuade people to take part in research.

Conclusions

It is, of course, unfortunate that ethical committees are needed to ensure that the consent of research participants is valid and that researchers behave in an ethical fashion. The main ethical principles – non-maleficence (do no harm), beneficence (do positive good), autonomy (show respect for rights of self-determination), and justice (treat people fairly) – should be uppermost in the minds of researchers and should at all times guide their behaviour. Focusing on the researcher's duties is fundamental. All too often the emphasis in discussions of the ethics of research is on the state of mind of the research participant. Are the participants competent to consent; have they understood the information they have been given; have they been given enough information to help them make a sound decision; and is their consent voluntary? There has been a welcome shift in recent years from the state of mind of the potential research participant to the conduct of the researcher and the bodies that control and monitor the activities of researchers, but all too often seeking ethics committee approval is seen as a bureaucratic hurdle to be overcome, rather than an opportunity to reflect on the ethical aspects of a piece of research.

References

Beauchamp, T.L. (1991) Competence, in M.A. Gardner Cuter and E.E. Shelp (eds) *Competency: A Study of Informal Competency Determinations in Primary Care*, pp. 49–77. London: Kluwer Academic Publishers.

Belmont Report (1978) *Ethical Principles and Guidelines for the Protection of Human Subjects of Research*. Publication No. OS 78-0012. Washington, DC: United States Department of Health, Education and Welfare.

Brazier, M. (1987) *Medicine, Patients and the Law*. London: Penguin Books.

Canterbury v. Spence [1972] 464 F.2s772, 780.

Downie, R.S. and Calman, K.C. (1987) *Healthy Respect: Ethics in Health Care*, Chapter 18. London: Faber and Faber.

Dubler, N.N. (1985) Some legal and moral issues surrounding informed consent for treatment and research involving the cognitively impaired elderly, in M.B. Kapp, H. E. Pies and A. E. Doudera (eds) *Legal and Ethical Aspects of Health Care for the Elderly*, pp. 247–57. Ann Arbor, MI: Health Administration Press.

Dworkin, G. (1987) Law and medical experimentation of embryos, children and others with limited legal capacity, *Monash University Law Review*, 13: 189–208.

Gilbert, C., Fulford, K.W.M. and Parker, C. (1989) Diversity in the practice of district ethics committees, *British Medical Journal*, 299: 1437–9.

Harris, J. (1985) *The Value of Life: An Introduction to Medical Ethics*, pp. 226–8. London: Routledge and Kegan Paul.

Kapp, M.B. and Bigot, A. (1985) *Geriatrics and the Law*, pp. 171–84. New York, NY: Springer Publishing Company.

Kennedy, I. (1988) The law and ethics of informed consent and randomized controlled trials, in *Treat Me Right: Essays in Medical Law and Ethics*. Oxford: Clarendon Press.

McLean, S.A.M. (1989) *A Patient's Right to know*. Aldershot: Dartmouth.

McLean, S. and Maher, G. (1983) Experimentation, in *Medicine, Morals and the Law*. Aldershot: Gower.

Makarushka, J. and McDonald, R. (1979) Informed consent, research and geriatric patients: the responsibility of institutional review committees, *The Gerontologist*, 19: 61.

Neuberger, J. (1992) *Ethics and Health Care: The Role of Research Ethics Committees in the United Kingdom*. London: Kings Fund Institute.

Ratzan, R.M. (1980) 'Being old makes you different': the ethics of research with elderly participants, *Hastings Center Report*, 10: 32–42.

Rights and Legal Protection Sub-Committee, Scottish Action on Dementia (1992) *Consent to Research*, Volume 2. Edinburgh: Scottish Action on Dementia (now Alzheimer's Scotland Action on Dementia).

Sidaway v. Board of Governors of the Bethlem Royal and the Maudsley Hospital [1984] 2 W.L.R. 778.

Thompson, I.E., French, K., Melia, K.M. *et al.* (1981) Research ethics committees in Scotland, *British Medical Journal*, 282: 718–20.

Waters, W.E. (1980) Role of the public in monitoring research with human participants, in *Issues in Research with Human Participants*, Part 6, NIH Publication No. 80-1858. Washington, DC: National Institutes of Health.

14

The role of older people in social research

Sheila Peace

Introduction: why involve older people in research?

The rhetoric of participation is everywhere. For several decades people have been encouraged to take part in the democratic process of our communities from being a school governor to collecting for a local charity to canvassing for a political party, and some people have always wanted to be, and have had the opportunity to be, more involved than others. But this is also true of those people who 'want to find out' and understand their world. Knowledge is everywhere and participation in knowledge production is developing.

The lay voice is becoming increasingly mainstreamed within every avenue of society and this can depend on how intimately they are involved as service users. In some cases people are involved in service evaluation and change; in other cases they are part of the process of consultation and decision making (see Figure 14.1). Involvement is becoming visible and everyday experts meet with academic, professional and managerial experts. They provide different views that may be viewed as having a different value.

Service users may be seen as a special group of people. While we are all service users in some ways, particular groups, for a whole range of reasons, will have become users of services, particularly health, social care and housing services, in order to survive. Inequalities that impact in later life will mean that many will be older people. They may not be the same kind of user as a younger person with a disability or mental health problem,

Advisory groups
Advocates/information givers
Campaigners/direct action
Consultative groups
Forums
Lay experts
Networks
Research respondents
User-led services
User panels
User/pensioners' groups

Figure 14.1   Forms of involvement in consultation and decision making
Source: Developed with reference to Peace 1999; Carter and Beresford 2000: vii

although they may suffer similar labels of vulnerability due to age, gender, ethnicity and social class.

Consequently, older people have become one of the groups whose views are increasingly sought, with their participation ranging from being any 'person on the street' to 'the user of specific services'. Views are being canvassed within the wider recognition of the need to understand an ageing society and as part of the modernization of services. The views that are heard may have different purposes – from action to participation to response – and the level of involvement may be chosen or requested. There is a difference between research participant and user participant.

What we do know is that there have been developments in research participation especially over the last thirty years. In 'hearing the user voice' we have moved from the muted tones reported by Booth (1983), for example, talking of the invisibility of older people living in residential care settings to the more authoritative input of people taking part in NISW's *Shaping Our Lives* (1998). We have moved from the early discussion of the usability of research in the field of ageing outlined by Osbourn and Willcocks (1990) to learning more about *involvement* such as:

- the older people taking part in the participative research projects funded by the Averil Osbourn Fund (Warren and Maltby 2000);
- the 28 pilot projects of the Better Government for Older People Forums (Hayden and Boaz 2000);
- Age Concern's *Debate of the Age* (Age Concern 1999),

and the more formalized development by funding bodies such as the Joseph Rowntree Foundation's Older People's Programme Steering Group and the Older People's Advisory Committee for the ESRC's Growing Older Programme.

- Encourage and value the contribution of participants.
- Seek the views of local people on a wide range of issues.
- Seek to involve a broad spread of people from the target populations.
- Choose appropriate consultation methods for the topic and the target group.
- Invest in consultation.
- Follow up consultations with feedback and action.
- Set in place mechanisms for ongoing consultation and involvement.

Figure 14.2 Good practice principles for consultation from the evaluation of the Better Government for Older People pilots
Source: Hayden and Boaz 2000: 3

People are being consulted in various ways as individuals and as groups and good practice principles have been developed concerning representation, methods, feedback and maintenance (Figure 14.2). But still there is a need to understand how the evidence that is communicated evolves and what the relationship is between consultation, participation and research (Peace 1999; Carter and Beresford 2000; Hayden and Boaz 2000).

We could say that all of these principles for consultation relate to different aspects of practitioner research but they might also be seen to relate in very specific ways to the different qualitative and quantitative methodological approaches to which this book has drawn our attention.

Here my concern is with the *role* of older people within research and taken in its broadest sense this means anyone involved in the search for knowledge. So, on the one hand, a great deal of research related to ageing involves people who are participants of services, while on the other, they are everyday participants of social networks, family formation, generators of historical knowledge, users of space etc. Because of this dual role as people who are more, or less, defined as users, this chapter draws upon a range of literature to inform the discussion concerning the role of older people in research.

To start, then, let us consider whether there is a difference between the *lay participant activist* and the *research respondent* who just happened to be in when the researcher called and they met the needs of the sample. Are people 'informants' or people 'with the knowledge', or are they participants who have questions to ask, or all of these? To try to answer these questions it is useful to think about the roles and relationships between research workers and older people.

Roles and relationships

In Figure 14.3 I have used the research discourse to try to identify the different roles that older people and others (who may be research workers,

Traditional research worker roles	Older person's roles	Additional roles for research worker
Proposal receiver/ developer	Funder Originator/s of idea/project	Facilitator/listener/translator
Fieldworker • recruiter • interviewer • observer • group facilitator • recorder • reader	Fieldworker • interviewer • observer • listener • recorder	Teacher/trainer • helper/co-worker • facilitator/ • negotiator/ • knower
Data preparer	Advisor/commentator Participant • respondent • knower	Listener/translator Fieldworker • interviewer/observer/ • analyst/knower
Analyst • reader • categorizer • interpreter • computer user • statistician	Analyst • reader • interpreter • categorizer • computer user • statistician	Teacher/helper • co-analyst/ • knower Feedback giver
Disseminator • writer • speaker • teacher • communicator • feedback giver	User/writer Disseminator Activist	Provider • originator of usable information/advocate Disseminator

Figure 14.3   Changing roles in research

practitioners or policy makers) may have in the broad area of enquiry called research. In the first column is the traditional research worker role that has developed during the past century as different research epistemologies have evolved. To a certain extent a level of control is with research workers and their colleagues who are part of various institutional structures, academic and otherwise. They have a range of roles which relate to methodology, data collection, analysis and dissemination.

The second column takes as its starting point the older person, who may or may not be the subject of the research, but who could be engaged in the process from funder, to originator of the idea, to interpreter of the data, to conveyor of the findings. The level of involvement may lead to a more or less participatory position and to varying levels of power between the different parties. The diversity of roles enables us to understand why some older people may not want, or have the ability and/or opportunity, to act in these ways. However, in reflecting on the greater involvement of older people, we can also outline additional roles for those employed as paid research workers, and in the third column I expand their role. Here they come to need a breadth of skills that may redefine their job and involves them acting more often as a trainer of others, facilitator and negotiator. Both parties need to share their knowledge and, which ever intermix of involvement is adopted, a partnership is created and a degree of shared research management may evolve.

Depending on the research framework and tradition adopted, the role of the research worker may be seen in a number of different ways, and a far more traditional role may be valued by the organization in which a researcher is employed than the one he or she may wish to develop. The challenge for the research worker may be to hold traditional and additional roles at the same time while trying to shift the acceptance of change. Having set up this alternative framework for research, are there ways of thinking about approaches to research that would be helpful to this discussion?

Research paradigms

The philosophical climate of research is ever changing and encompasses the positivist scientific tradition which sees research evidence as based on the statistical understanding of probability to provide evidence; deliberations regarding the interplay of quantitative and qualitative research methodology and material; methods of understanding narrative biographical and life course material; and participatory research, developments in action research and the 'emancipatory paradigm'. If, as has been suggested, the experiences of certain types of research in the field of ageing may be becoming more participatory, can we learn from similar developments within other fields of study?

In discussing the involvement of older service users within research and evaluation, Barnes and Walker (1996) reflected on the development of consumerism and began by looking at features of *bureaucratic organizations* that are service-centred, top-down, power-concentrated, relatively inflexible and dependent on inputs (see also Brown 2000). The features of these organizations are outlined below (Figure 14.4), and I have set alongside them components of the *scientific, positivist* research paradigm, where, although from a totally different discourse, there are broad commonalities in terms of linearity and authority with objectivity underpinning this research tradition.

Does the identification of similarities between the structure of organizational systems and research thinking mean that alternatives need to be

Bureaucratic service organization	*Positivist research*
Top-down	Theory-driven, hypothesis-testing
Power-concentrated	Quantification, numbers
Defensive	Probability
Conservative	Objectivity
Input-oriented	Researcher-distanced
	Theory-derived

Figure 14.4   Features of bureaucratic organizations and positivist research

Source: developed with reference to Barnes and Walker 1996

based within a non-positivist, qualitative or ethnographic research frame that recognizes the value of subjectivity? This has certainly been a feature of feminist research and work in the fields of ethnicity, community development and disability. While *participatory research* may be the overarching description of this work, they are also called *emancipatory* and *empowering* research models (Roberts 1990; Stanley and Wise 1983; Hart and Bond 1995; Barnes and Walker 1996; Stone and Priestley 1996). These terms involve issues of personal development and partnership between the researchers and the researched alongside recognition of difference.

While research perspectives may span the continuum of objectivity and subjectivity coming together methodologically through triangulation (Fielding and Fielding 1986; Layder 1993), here I utilize the 'ideal types'. At one extreme the research process may evolve from an issue where a hypothesis is developed which can then be tested through using various research techniques with a research population. Such questions may be couched within a theoretical framework. The research subjects may be chosen randomly or through stratification and a distance is maintained between subject and researcher. Analysis of data will result in the hypothesis being rejected or accepted. This is a linear process which Stanley and Wise (1983), from a feminist tradition, called 'hygienic research' and which rarely features in reality. Their discussion of the development of 'feminist social science research' presented a challenge to positivism and stressed the importance of researcher involvement. They commented on the impact that being objective may have on the performance of the researcher:

'Within positivism and naturalism this usually means that we present our work as scholarly and detached from what we have conducted research on. It may now be all right to be involved, committed even, but we must necessarily preserve 'scholarly detachment'.

(Stanley and Wise 1983: 155)

Empowering research	Emancipatory research – disability movement	Action research
Personal development/ control of 'knowers'	Control rests with 'knowers'	Problem-focused
Equal balance of power	Surrender of objectivity	Context-specific
Develops partnership	Linked to political action	Involves change intervention
Supported within wider system	Brings about change	Aims at improvement/ involvement
Maintains ownership of responsibilities	Research skills utilized	Cyclic process – research, action, evaluation
Supported by adequate resources	Interlink personal/political individual/collective	Participation through research
Collective as well as individual process	Recent recognition of methodological plurality	Future-oriented

Figure 14.5   Characteristics of emancipatory, empowering and action research approaches

Note: These characteristics have been brought together from readings within the fields of disability, social care, ageing and health

And they stressed the importance of the personal within research:

> Basic to feminism is that 'the personal is the political'. We suggest that this insistence on the crucial importance of the personal must also include an insistence on the importance, and also the presence, of the personal within research experiences as much as within any other experiences.
>
> (1983: 158)

These understandings have more recently been developed by those undertaking research in disability. Figure 14.5 sets out aspects of the *'emancipatory paradigm'* supported by those within the disability movement who adhere to the social model of disability where disability is seen as 'socially constructed and culturally produced' (Oliver 1990), a product of disabling environments and attitudes. Writers working within this model have developed a new grounding for research that is underpinned by a philosophy setting particular parameters around the research process, and these ideas could relate to the new roles for older people outlined in Figure 14.3.

In this case the original thinking surrounding research ideas lies with disabled people as the people who 'know', who remain in control of the process and utilize the skills of researchers. In this way the power base is to be up-ended. Another central feature is to bring about change and develop action. There is a central commitment to a particular way of thinking about an oppressed position and, because of this, research is seen as political as well as personal. In terms of research methodology this has led to the dominance of qualitative methods although there has been a more recent recognition of the value of mixed approaches enabling an interface between the individual and the collective (Stone and Priestley 1996). It could be argued that gerontological research, while recognizing the impact of the social construction of ageing, is not driven by such a philosophical paradigm and encompasses a wide variety of perspectives.

However, some forms of research are more likely to be seen as *empowering* than others. Barnes and Walker (1996) use the term empowering research to focus on service-user involvement and contrast this view with the bureaucratic model outlined in Figure 14.4. Here *participation* in research leads to forms of empowerment. There is an emphasis on partnership with the coming together of research workers and 'knowers' to share their expertise, encourage personal development and utilize skills of negotiation (see Barnes 1993). They also recognize the need for resources and support in order to move from participation into action.

The final example from participative research mentioned here is that of *action research* developed in social psychology, education, community development, nursing and management which Hart and Bond discuss as 'generating knowledge about a social system while, at the same time trying to change it' (1995: 13). This type of research could also be called *practitioner research* where the research role is steered by those with a practice role. While the ability to bring about change is central, the focus comes from a specific problem and is part of a collective process that is developmental and where all the parties are part of the process of change which is ongoing and cyclical. Some of the approaches outlined here have common characteristics around participation, empowerment, shared expertise, the link between the personal and the political and the importance of outcome in terms of implementation and change.

Reflections from researchers

In discussing these methods writers have commented on their experiences as research workers, separating out their views on the value of the process for the participants and the value for themselves as researchers based in academic organizations or other bodies.

While they may empathize with the people who give the research information and wish to develop participatory approaches, they also recognize that it may lead the participants to experience conflict and tensions. The contradictions experienced by researchers, who may or may not be practitioners, in belonging to 'at least' two or three camps is fundamental. Where people's views are couched within a very particular philosophy which has specific implications for them as disempowered people it can be very hard to vocalize the pressures that may surround the research worker. Stone and Priestley (1996) discuss two studies in which they have been involved as doctoral students working with disabled people, and the constraints faced by researchers. They describe what they call a 'tug-of-war':

> Regardless of the commitment to the emancipatory paradigm, the researcher is required to bow in several directions: to research councils and to academic peers, to disabled people and their organisations. The researcher both acts and is acted upon within these power relationships.
> (Stone and Priestley 1996: 708)

Tensions may ensue: for example, surrendering overall control of the research, and the expectations of the academic community in terms of research professionalism and research dissemination. This raises issues relating to research funding, personal employment, contract working and status, and may engender insecurity in these areas. In many ways researchers may experience similar feelings of disempowerment to those of lay 'experts'. They may be aware of the need for a partnership within the research process but recognize problems surrounding research ownership related to research funding and issues of accountability over dissemination and implementation. Dissemination to a range of parties including ongoing feedback needs to be valued and recognized in research proposals. Goodley and Moore (2000) illustrate how research material developed pictorially with people with learning difficulties can be disseminated in different ways and challenge the dominant modes of research production. There is a need for other innovative methods.

However, for those working within disability research there is also a recognition that not every disabled person will necessarily accept similar philosophical perspectives or approaches which do not allow for diverse understandings. One set of disadvantages may be replaced by another, as shown by this comment concerning the feelings of some research participants:

> It is evident that individual disabled service users may sometimes feel as alienated by the politicized nature of disabled people's organisations as they do by state welfare bureaucracies. Devolving control over the research production to a local coalition of disabled people may seem a straightforward means of achieving accountability but it may do little to directly empower individual research participants in the process.
> (Stone and Priestley 1996: 710)

In this case, the researchers chose to publicize their research as theory-driven and therefore they were taking an emancipatory approach. Consequently, they saw their work as having a wider impact. The basis from which the researchers are working will therefore affect the consequences. But it should be acknowledged that the peer group of the researched can also exert pressures.

While not denying that in any field there will be people willing and able to learn or share the skills of the paid researcher in order to have control over the process of research, this may not always be possible, desired or advisable. Walmsley (2001) discusses what the term *inclusive research* means in working with people with learning difficulties, showing the way in which both parties need each other as allies so that if one party cannot undertake an aspect of a project, another party can. For example, this may be in relation to: a research skill; theoretical development; control over the purpose of the research; or the development of questions. In this way theory and action may develop in parallel.

The views of these researchers enable us to appreciate something of the researchers' experiences and some of the issues raised through the involvement of different constituencies. Research involving older people needs further unpacking (Peace 1999).

Examples of studies: some key issues

In acknowledging the potential of intermixing roles, a number of issues begin to take on more importance within the research arena with implications for all forms of methodology. Here I use examples from different studies to look at representation and skills.

Representation

The type of research being undertaken will have a direct bearing on the people involved. Those being asked to respond to a research question in a *survey* by being chosen through random, stratified or purposive samples will have been approached by the researchers in definable ways and will be seen as representative of a general population or as a person with specific characteristics. Older people taking part in *participative research*, or *practitioner research* will also have certain characteristics. Their unifying feature may be that they are service users, but they may also be people of a certain age, gender or ethnicity, chosen in a specific way. This is not to decry the approach but to recognize and identify differentials within similar roles.

Barnes and Walker (1996) were able to consider these aspects of their empowering model in relation to their evaluative work with the Fife User Panels Project. These panels started in 1992 originally to involve older service users in community care planning but they later evolved to enable older people to participate in influencing other forms of policy implementation. The representativeness of different types of people in such groups is often questioned. Barnes and Walker (1996) give this account of the development of the panels, which indicates their diversity and also demonstrates that the approach does not appeal to everyone, sets criteria, and does not include some frail older people:

> Potential panel members are identified by social work and health services providers, through ACS networks, and by existing panel members. Criteria for membership are that people are users or potential users of community services, normally (though not exclusively) living on their own and over 75 years of age. It was decided that the model proposed would not be appropriate for a mixed group involving people with dementia. A total of 62 people were nominated and agreed to become panel members during the first three years of the project. Another 28 were nominated but decided that it was not for them. The youngest member was 67, the oldest 93. The average age was 82, but the biggest single group were aged between 86 and 90. Men were considerably outnumbered: only eight men became panel members in this period: 55 of the panel members lived alone and 49 were widowed; seven had never been married. By definition, all the panel members experienced one or more health problems, or were disabled. Only six were not in receipt of aids to daily living, and only two were not in regular receipt of health or social care services.
>
> (Barnes and Walker 1996: 387)

The views of panel members were gained mostly through small group work around specific topics and innovative methods such as games were used. These may not be seen as traditional 'research tools' but served their purpose. Members' views were sometimes sought on wider research design and the development of questionnaires, while on other occasions their work would have a direct practical outcome such as a 14-point 'Good Hospital Discharge' checklist. It was not the responsibility of the panels to do their own research but to respond and innovate through their discussions. They were not seen as 'representative' but 'typical of others':

> Panel members were invited to join the panels to speak from their own experiences and on their own behalf. They were not expected to 'represent' other older people either statistically or democratically. Nevertheless, those invited to join were considered to be typical of other older people in similar circumstances (Barnes et al. 1994). One of the rules of the panels was that project workers would not advocate on behalf of individuals. Panel members recognised that participation was not a direct route to securing services for themselves, but that through the collective expression of their voices, they could contribute to service improvements which would benefit older people generally.
>
> (Barnes and Walker 1996: 389)

Change may have developed through this process but responsibility and accountability did not rest with the panel members. An evaluation of the panels has shown that for some, but not all, membership led to personal development, if not a wider sense of participation. Yet, while empowering for some, others' personal circumstances, such as declining health, over-shadowed their involvement, leading to less engagement.

These comments are indicative of other studies where certain groups of older people have been under-represented. Meg Bond tells her 'story of the steps taken by older people, carers and workers in what may be described as a demonstration project to improve local institutional and community care' (Hart and Bond 1995: 127). In this piece of work she was employed as a jointly funded social worker attached to a doctor's practice with the role of aiming to reach older people with health and illness problems who may have social needs but would not turn to social services. Her story tells first of the development of a Community Forum of multidisciplinary pro-fessionals which developed a Special Interest Group for Elderly People which shared experiences and information. This professional development led to a decision to invite local older people to join them for a discussion of growing older within their particular neighbourhood. The workers were conscious of the people who never get invited to join and this is how the membership is described:

> We put considerable thought into who should be invited and how. We knew from our discussions of Christmas treats that some people got all the invitations and some none, and we knew from our session on 'the invisible elderly' that we were only in touch with a minority of pen-sioners. Moreover, many of those we knew were frail and housebound with failing sight and hearing. How could we enable them to take part fully – to hear and be heard? Our series of earlier meetings stood us in good stead to deal with these dilemmas because we had reached some understanding of the problems facing older people, and we had est-ablished a firm shared commitment to open up a dialogue with them. Between us we were in touch with a cross section of older people spanning an age range of some thirty or so years, including some who were fit, bed-bound, supported, isolated, council tenants, owner occu-piers, in receipt of means-tested benefits and members of local pen-sioners' groups. We decided that a personal approach was more likely to produce a response than a written invitation or posters advertising a public meeting.
>
> (Hart and Bond 1995: 135)

Interestingly, in a later evaluation Meg Bond comments on the relation-ship of the process undertaken to the types of people involved:

The open planning format:

- includes stalwarts who are pensioners and members of local pensioners' groups;
- includes a number of older and younger helpers who come as volunteers and/or Age Concern members and who have been drawn in because of their skills and interests e.g. as handicraft experts through the Women and Health group and residents' association and as volunteer drivers and fund raisers;
- has lost some of its early members, perhaps because information about planning meetings has usually been passed on verbally rather than formally in writing by a secretary;
- lacks male pensioners;
- lacks a direct input from frailer housebound people;
- has failed to draw in older people from the black and Asian communities;
- lacks a regular input from the domiciliary health services.

(Hart and Bond 1995: 142)

It is true that some people will always get involved but it is important to consider the degree to which people wish to engage or disengage throughout life and as they get older. For some it will be a case of 'never having been asked'; for others energy levels or particular impairments may work against involvement; while some people are just not interested. How far the diversity of older people is recognized relates to issues of sampling and, as noted, participative approaches may fail to meet certain quotas.

The difference in response may also vary in terms of the type of research method within which people are asked to participate. Levels of group or individual participation can always form part of the research process. At one end there are the practical issues of inclusion which relate to recording data, and the need for new tools within methodologies may be needed. But other factors are more personal: joining a focus group may be less threatening to some than keeping a diary, but for others an in-depth interview may be far more rewarding than having your behaviour observed.

Issues of representation are still open to debate. How far are the views of different groups and individuals generalizable for others? What is the evidence they produce and how might this inform practice? In one corner we may have statistical reliability while in the other detailed analysis of individual biographical narrative.

The research skills of older people

If older people may have greater involvement in research – whatever the aspect of participation – there will be a need to broaden the roles of all parties. Some people will need to acquire new skills and others to reuse skills that they may not have used for some time. While some people will lack the confidence to be involved directly, others may be coping with specific physical difficulties regarding hearing, seeing and moving which need to be addressed to enable involvement. These issues all need to be recognized and built into the research design as they demand extra time and extra resources.

For example, far more is now being discovered about the well-being and personhood of people with dementia (Kitwood and Bredin 1992; Kitwood 1997; Bamford and Bruce 2000), and their inclusion shows a need for the development of the skill of *listening*. In discussing her interviews with four older women with dementia in an attempt to consider their subjective experience, Gillian Proctor (2001) used a Voice Relational Method to understand different ways in which the women were talking. The research method also enabled the researcher to look at the issue of power within the researcher/participant relationship. By spending time with the participants she was able to take their words back to them, read them to them, and further the discussions. In this way the process was reflexive, creating a dialogue through the researcher developing skills that enable the older women to participate. As she says: 'the women seemed pleased that what they spoke about was taken seriously and their views were considered' (2001: 374).

Research workers and funding bodies are beginning to be aware of these demands (Peace 1999). *Administrative support* may become a worker's role. Elizabeth Mosse and Pat Thornton, in talking about an advisory group of older people set up to assist a project aimed at identifying opportunities for older people to have a say in planning and evaluating community care services, show how this became a learning experience for everyone. No one was an expert, power sharing had to evolve and people needed to feel valued:

> Elizabeth commented that no-one knew what was happening at the beginning but they gradually gained confidence to discuss issues between themselves. The atmosphere was good. The researchers organised transport and there were refreshments. It was not overawing. It was agreed that the researchers should do all the paperwork – agendas, minutes, etc. and they were kept well-informed on the progress of the research and how the fieldwork was going. They met one of the groups in the field.
>
> The question was raised as to whether they should have been doing the fieldwork. There was no direct answer here and it depended very much on people's motivation and the level at which they wished to participate. It had not been expected of them in this instance. However, Elizabeth commented that once they had been given practical tasks to do together such as work on the questionnaire, the group felt valued. Although there was an underlying feeling that the researchers might not take on board their ideas. Personally doing the summary findings had been 'demanding work but well worth doing'.
>
> (Peace 1999: 8)

As Walmsley (2001) stated, there is a need for 'knowers' and researchers to become allies and assist each other, views also discussed by Cormie and Warren (2001: 41) in their guidelines for running discussion groups with older people.

In Figure 14.3 I identified *teaching/training* as roles for researchers while participants developed new skills. This role can relate to various aspects of the research process such as interviewing or analysing data, and the level of training may vary from a few days to several weeks, encompassing issues relating to coping with cultural difference and physical impairment. As this member of the Lewisham Older Women's Network comments when talking about analysing data from their health survey, support and patience are essential:

> We had got our data and now it had to be analysed both quantitatively and qualitatively. Maureen was the organiser for the initial process and she met us at a variety of venues in Lewisham. Some were big and we had plenty of room for putting our papers around. Some were very cramped. She had great patience because we didn't always get the same people coming to every meeting. So it meant going back again and starting with new people that day and telling them what we've done the day before, or time before. But everyone had great patience and everyone was enjoying it. And we got on and finally we managed to do that part of it.
>
> (Peace 1999: 20)

Some projects offer extensive training – a project run jointly by Lancaster University and Counsel and Care for the Elderly on Housing Decisions has employed older people as researchers and ran a 20-week Research Methods Course.[1] In reflecting on this development the researchers have commented on issues such as the need to build in sufficient time for training and preparation and the complication of open access to potential interviewers, some of whom needed to be carefully monitored (Holland, personal communication, 2001).

Another recent study looking at the housing, care and supportive needs of visually impaired older people (Hanson *et al.* 2001) also involves older people interviewing 400 other older people. Here the researchers are training members of the University of the Third Age who have volunteered to be interviewers. We need to learn more about what people make of this experience. Researcher John Percival spoke to one of the female interviewers, who herself had some visual impairment, and who had this to say about the experience:

Q: Why did you agree to do this interviewing?
A: I think because of getting older myself, and I've had physical disabilities myself, and I thought I wanted to get an idea of what older

people are dealing with and what is available to them. Also, I care about what happens to older people and thought I could help them in some way.

Q: What do you think are the advantages and disadvantages of older people interviewing other older people?

Mary immediately answered that the big advantage is that 'they [older interviewers] have empathy with the older person'. Mary could not so easily think of disadvantages, but eventually concluded that one would be if the older interviewer fails to carry out a sensitive interview because s/he is 'swayed by their own problems, their own situation'. That is to say, the older interviewer is preoccupied by her own difficulties to such an extent that these dominate conversation and inhibit listening to the interviewee.

Q: What do you have to learn to do this work?

A: An acceptance of others' views, of different views from your own, and not to make quick judgements, to think you know what the [older] person is really like and what they have to go through.

Mary went on to say that sometimes it can be difficult to maintain an absolutely objective stance, particularly when the interviewee comes across as aggressive, fearful or lonely. She concluded that you have to learn and accept but not give your opinion.

(Source: Personal correspondence with John Percival 2001)

While this is only one experience it does indicate how personal understanding can have implications in terms of the objectivity and subjectivity of the older person as research worker. The role of older people as research fieldworkers may influence empathy between players, although age difference, gender, ethnicity and personality will also have a bearing on relationships between other research workers and their respondents.

Nevertheless, extending involvement and developing partnership can be questioned within the research world (Hammersley 1992). Not everyone agrees with the appropriateness of skill sharing. Some people may be thought to be trained to do a certain task and more detached in their application of research methods. While there may be a desire to develop greater equity within the research there is also a recognition that the skills of the research worker may mean that in certain situations they have more power than the research knower, although one cannot move forwards without the other (see Maynard 1994).

Issues of validity

This discussion shows that variation in types of representation and methodological approach will influence the value attached to the evidence.

Participative approaches and practitioner research may lead to action around specific issues but they may, or may not, be relevant to other situations. Beyond the specific sphere of service intervention, the researcher will play an important role in establishing the validity of data, often crucial in order to establish a strength of argument especially where there is an interplay of various sources (Kellaher *et al.* 1990). In developing more innovative research approaches it will be important to bring different traditions and disciplines together so that evidence may encompass both broad-based samples and individual depth. There also needs to be an understanding of the different ways in which research findings may be valued that is both immediate, leading to action, and long-term and cumulative, leading to theoretical development.

Conclusions

This chapter began by making the point that potentially all older people could become involved in the research process and that they do not have to be service users whose participation is being encouraged through user involvement. In broadening this perspective it is apparent that there are many roles that older people may take with consequent knock-on effects for other paid researchers. The development of participative research is relatively new and its influence within the panoply of wider movements and discussions – concerning user involvement, evidence-based practice, debate about the value attributed to objective and subjective data, and what is meant by excellence – is still to be charted. For those researching ageing and later life, the role of older people within this process will vary depending on the issue, the context, the funding and, fundamentally, the purpose being served by the research process.

Acknowledgements

With many thanks to the following researchers who have reviewed and contributed to this chapter: Dorothy Atkinson, Tim Clements, Caroline Holland, Leonie Kellaher, Anne Jamieson, John Percival.

Notes

1 The research methods course is now being run in two locations: Lancaster University's Department of Continuing Education and London's National Institute of Social Work (November 2001).

References

Age Concern England (1999) *Debate of the Age*. London: Age Concern England.

Bamford, C. and Bruce, E. (2000) Defining the outcomes of community care: the perspectives of older people with dementia and their carers, *Ageing and Society*, 20(5): 543–70.

Barnes, M. (1993) Introducing new stakeholders – user and research interests in evaluative research. A discussion of methods used to evaluate the Birmingham Community Care Special Action Project, *Policy and Politics*, 24(1): 47–58.

Barnes, M. and Walker, A. (1996) Consumerism versus empowerment: a principled approach to the involvement of older service users, *Policy and Politics*, 24(4): 375–93.

Booth, T. (1983) Residents' views, rights and institutional care, in M. Fisher (ed.) *Speaking of Clients*, Social Services Monographs: Research into Practice. Sheffield: Joint Unit for Social Services Research/Community Care, University of Sheffield.

Brown, H. (2000) Challenges from service-users, in A. Brechin, H. Brown and M.A. Eby (eds) *Critical Practice in Health and Social Care*. London: Sage Publications.

Carter, T. and Beresford, P. (2000) *Age and Change: Models of Involvement for Older People*. York: Joseph Rowntree Foundation.

Cormie, J. and Warren, L. (2001) *Working with Older People. Guidelines for Running Discussion Groups and Influencing Practice*. Bristol: Policy Press.

Everitt, A., Hardiker, P., Littlewood, J. and Mullender, A. (1992) *Applied Research for Better Practice*. London: Macmillan.

Fielding, N. and Fielding, J. (1986) *Linking Data*. Qualitative Research Methods Series, 4. London: Sage Publications.

Goodley, D. and Moore, M. (2000) Doing disability research: activist lives and the academy, *Disability and Society*, 15(6): 861–82.

Hammersley, M. (1992) *What's Wrong with Ethnography?* London: Routledge.

Hanson, J., Johnson, M., Percival, J. and Zako, R. (2001) Ongoing research study, 'The Housing, Care and Support Needs of Older Visually Impaired People', funded by the Gift of Thomas Pocklington.

Hart, E. and Bond, M. (1995) *Action Research for Health and Social Care: A Guide to Practice*. Buckingham: Open University Press.

Hayden, C. and Boaz, A. (2000) *Making a Difference*. Better Government for Older People Evaluation Report. Coventry: Local Government Centre, University of Warwick.

Kellaher, L., Peace, S. and Willcocks, D. (1990) Triangulating data, in S. Peace (ed.) *Researching Social Gerontology*. London: Sage Publications.

Kitwood, T. (1997) *Dementia Reconsidered: The Person Comes First*. Buckingham: Open University Press.

Kitwood, T. and Bredin, K. (1992) Towards a theory of dementia care: personhood and well-being, *Ageing and Society*, 12: 269–87.

Layder, D. (1993) *New Strategies in Social Research*. London: Polity Press.

Maynard, M. (1994) Methods, practice and epistemology: the research debate about feminism and research, in M. Maynard and J. Purvis (eds) *Researching Women's Lives from a Feminist Perspective*. London: Taylor & Francis.

Morris, J. (1992) Personal and political: a feminist perspective on researching physical disability, *Disability, Handicap and Society*, 7(2): 157–66.

National Institute for Social Work (1998) *Shaping Our Lives*. London: NISW.

Osborn, A. and Willcocks, D. (1990) Making research useful and usable, in S.M. Peace (ed.) *Researching Social Gerontology: Concepts, Methods and Issues*. London: Sage Publications.

Peace, S. (ed.) (1999) *Involving Older People in Research: 'An Amateur Doing the Work of a Professional?'* London: Centre for Policy on Ageing/Centre for Ageing and Biographical Studies.

Proctor, G. (2001) Listening to older women with dementia: relationships, voices and power, *Disability and Society*, 16(3): 361–76.

Roberts, H. (ed.) (1990) *Doing Feminist Research*. London: Routledge.

Stanley, L. and Wise, S. (1983) *Breaking Out: Feminist Consciousness and Feminist Research*. London: Routledge and Kegan Paul.

Stone, E. and Priestley, M. (1996) Parasites, pawns and partners: disability research and the role of non-disabled researchers, *British Journal of Sociology*, 47(4): 699–716.

Thompson, N. (1995) *Theory and Practice in Health and Social Welfare*. Buckingham: Open University Press.

Walmsley, J. (2001) Normalisation, emancipatory research and inclusive research in learning disability, *Disability and Society*, 16(2): 187–205.

Warren, L. and Maltby, T. (2000) Averil Osbourn and participatory research, in A.M. Warnes, L. Warren and M. Nolan (eds) *Care Services for Later Life*. London: Jessica Kingsley Publishers.

15

The use of gerontological research in policy and practice

Mike Nolan
Jo Cooke

The creation of guidelines without significant attention to their application is clearly a sterile exercise.

(Davis and Taylor-Vaisey 1997: 415)

Ultimately evidence has no value to those that it affects unless it can be weighed properly by them.

(Walsh 1998: 92)

Introduction

Pearlin *et al.* (2001) contend that most researchers have a 'fervent hope' that their work will, in some way, make a difference. In other words, it is not sufficient that studies are published but rather results should be used to bring about desired change. The potential uses to which research can be put are many and it is not possible to consider all of them here. For example, Bengston *et al.* (1997) believe that gerontology is 'data rich but theory poor', citing the extensive empirical data that have been collected but bemoaning the fact that these have not resulted in more sophisticated theoretical insights. Clearly one very important 'use' to which research could be put in gerontology is to build more elegant theoretical accounts. We acknowledge and fully support such a position, but will not explore it further here. Instead we will focus on the more direct application of research to improve the health and social care that older people receive.

Osborn and Willcocks (1990) highlighted the importance of disseminating research widely, advocating that researchers disseminate their results so as to challenge attitudes and assumptions that limit choice and opportunity for older people. Such a position is as pertinent today as it was over a decade ago. However, we would like to extend the debate beyond dissemination in order to make research useful to, and ultimately usable by, not only policy makers and practitioners, but also older people themselves.

To do so it is important to consider how, and by whom, research might be useful in the context of developing improved services for older people. Rossi and Freeman (1993) suggest that research can be used in one of three broad ways:

- It can be *directly applied* in order to change current policy or practice.
- It can be used *conceptually* to challenge thinking or raise awareness of important issues relating to current policy/practice.
- It can be used *persuasively* to support the continuance of current policy/ practice, or to argue for change.

Others argue that research 'evidence' can be used to inform practice, purchasing, management or policy-making decisions (Muir-Gray 1997). Clearly, then, research may impact at several different levels, individually, organizationally and politically. Our focus in this chapter is on the barriers that exist to the 'transfer' of research to local health and social care contexts. Anderson *et al.* (1999) contend that relatively little attention has been given to how the academic and practice communities interact, arguing that research will not be used optimally until communication between these groups is improved. It is our intention to outline a framework illuminating the difficulties in applying research, and to offer some potential solutions. Ultimately, however, we believe that the most effective strategy is to reduce, and eventually eliminate, the 'distance' between both research and practice, and between differing forms of knowledge. The chapter will therefore conclude with a brief consideration of how this might be achieved.

Addressing the barriers to research utilization

The gap between research and practice is well known, and has been documented for some time (Needham 2000). However, the current emphasis on evidence-based practice has resulted in increased interest in how this gap might be reduced in health and social services (DoH 1996; Muir-Gray 1997). There is a realization that dissemination is not of itself sufficient to bring about change (Muir-Gray 1997; Kitson *et al.* 1998, NHS Centre for Reviews and Dissemination 1999; Hughes *et al.* 2000), and that utilizing research in practice requires a multifaceted approach (Le May 1999) which addresses a complex interplay of factors (James and Smith 1999) including the nature of the evidence; the values, beliefs and experiences of practitioners and users of services; and the context in which services are delivered. Therefore attention should not simply focus on dissemination, but rather on the development of comprehensive implementation strategies (Anderson *et al.* 1999).

Following an extensive consideration of the available literature, and a comparison of empirical studies exploring the barriers to the utilization of research among nurses in the UK, the USA, Sweden and Australia, Nolan *et al.* (1999) suggested that it is helpful to consider impediments to research use under five headings, comprising an alliteration of As. Each of these headings raises a number of questions and tensions that can be summarized as follows:

Availability: does the necessary research evidence exist? What counts as 'evidence' and who defines it as such?
Acceptability: is the available evidence of sufficient quality? Which criteria are used to judge quality and from whose perspective?
Awareness: are those who might use research aware of its existence? How is research disseminated and what status is given to differing means of dissemination?
Accessibility: is the research evidence accessible? Can those who might use research obtain it and, if they can, is it in a form that is readily understood?
Adoption: is the evidence widely adopted and used to produce change or to improve the current situation? What are the barriers to applying research and how might these be overcome?

These comprise a series of contingencies, with all five needing to be addressed if research is to be used optimally. Clearly research cannot be applied if it is not available, nor should it be applied if it does not comprise 'good' evidence. However, even if good-quality evidence is available it has little chance of being used if no one is aware of its existence, or cannot obtain it readily, or if it is presented in a form too complex to understand. Conversely, all of the above criteria might be met and evidence still not be applied. Even within the medical profession where there is the greatest availability of good-quality evidence, often in the form of explicit guidelines for practice, utilization remains problematic (Davis and Taylor-Vaisey 1997). A further appreciation of the complexities of the issues involved can be gained from a more detailed consideration of the five As above.

Is the evidence available?

The availability of evidence is limited by a number of factors, particularly existing research activity and capacity, especially in relation to social care

(Hughes *et al.* 2000). Iwaniec and Pinkerton (1998), for example, note that spending on research and development (R&D) comprises less than 1 per cent of service delivery costs, and a series of recent seminars highlighted the small and fragmented academic base for social work and social care research (see http://www.nisw.org.uk/tswr/; accessed 26 June 2002). Moreover, there is no real tradition of social work research and no strong academic leadership in the field (Iwaniec and Pinkerton 1998). This is exacerbated by the limited R&D infrastructure in local authorities and by the fact that research training rarely figures within social work preparation; nor is it seen as necessary for career progression (Smith *et al.* 2001). The effect of this was apparent in a study of social workers in Northern Ireland, which found that over half did not understand the varying research methodologies that were available but that 70 per cent wished to develop skills in this area (McCrystal 2000).

Medicine apart, similar circumstances limit the capacity for research within the health services, especially in nursing (Hunt 1996; Nolan *et al.* 1998). Therefore, despite the fact that the promotion of research in nursing has been a goal for over thirty years, significant barriers still remain (Hunt 1996; McSherry 1997; Dunn *et al.* 1998). Unless there is greater attention to capacity building in both health and social care the availability of research evidence will remain limited.

Is the evidence acceptable?

The current impetus towards evidence-based practice has its roots in medicine (Muir-Gray 1997) where there exists a widely accepted 'hierarchy' of evidence, at the top of which sits the 'randomized controlled trial' (RCT). So when Sackett *et al.* (1996: 71) define evidence-based medicine as 'the conscientious, explicit and judicious use of current best evidence in making decisions about individual patients', 'best evidence' is defined largely in terms of the gold standard of the RCT (Le May 1999). However, even within medicine, some see the primacy given to the RCT as a 'step too far' (Black 2001), and such tensions are more apparent within other disciplines providing health and social care.

Clarke (1999), for example, calls for a pluralistic and eclectic stance towards what constitutes evidence, while Walsh (1998) argues that valuing objective knowledge over subjective and social knowledge 'seriously disempowers' certain groups, especially patients.

The dominance of a medically orientated approach to research also exerts other detrimental effects. One obvious example is the type of research that receives funding, with the Department of Health (2001) confining research primarily to studies which produce 'generalizable' results. Although a more eclectic stance is now apparent, current definitions of what constitute 'best evidence' make it more difficult to obtain funding for qualitative studies.

This is ironic given the importance attached to capturing the 'experiences' of service users within recent policy initiatives such as the National Service Framework (NSF) for older people, and the need to understand not only the outcomes of care but also the context and processes within which care is delivered (Gomm 2000; Smith 2000). Many argue for the development of knowledge that is more context-specific (Brechin and Siddell 2000) but this is limited by the pervasive influence of biomedical perspectives and limited financial resources (Broad 1999).

There are calls for a strategic approach to promoting a diversity of social work research methodologies (Fisher 2000) including more interpretative and emancipatory approaches that result in differing, but possibly more relevant, forms of evidence (Brechin and Siddell 2000). This is especially important in light of the recent onus on incorporating a user perspective into the evidence base, which emphasizes the importance of building on the expertise which older people possess. Beresford (1999) proclaims that there is a need for 'a shift in power, in the context of knowledge and what counts as knowledge, with service users having more say in both'.

Whether research is deemed of acceptable quality therefore hinges largely on the definition of evidence adopted, and whose perspective is applied. However, acceptability is not simply a facet of the 'quality' of research, and if evidence is to be applied it also needs to be seen as relevant and plausible by those who might use it (Anderson *et al.* 1999). Topics which academics see as important may not 'grab' the imagination of practitioners and 'burning' issues for policy makers and planners may have similarly limited appeal (Adams *et al.* 1999; Broad 1999; Hughes *et al.* 2000). This suggests the need for a closer dialogue between researchers and practitioners (Anderson *et al.* 1999; Abbott and Hutchkins 2001) and between researchers and users (Hanley *et al.* 2000).

Awareness of research

High-quality research evidence may exist but it has little chance of being applied if there is limited awareness among practice communities. This has been problematic for at least two decades (Hunt 1981) and many novel ways of dissemination have been developed (see Box 15.1). Despite such initiatives, and the widespread availability of modern methods of communication, challenges remain. One way of promoting greater awareness of research has been through the development of systematic reviews and practice guidelines, and such developments continue through the National Institute for Clinical Excellence (NICE) in health care, and are being explored by the Social Care Institute for Excellence (SCIE) in social care. Once again, however, the evidence underpinning guidelines in health care is predicated almost exclusively on the gold standard of the RCT.

> **Box 15.1   A novel way to disseminate – audiotapes for practitioners on the move**
>
> Being mindful of appropriate ways to inform busy practitioners was the motivation behind using audiotapes as a way to disseminate research overviews undertaken by Research in Practice (RIP). RIP is a national membership organization comprising social service and voluntary bodies whose aim is to act as a catalyst for the use of evidence in services. They were aware that social workers spend up to 40 per cent of their work time in their cars, and suggested that summaries of research evidence delivered by audiotape could make better use of what otherwise might be wasted time. However, practitioners did not just use the tapes in cars, but at team meetings to stimulate lively debate on how the research messages could have an impact on practice. The evaluation of these tapes is currently underway and the findings are to be published.

Moreover, although dissemination is actively promoted it is not well funded relative to other aspects of the research process. Researchers are often unable to explore the development arm of R&D due to the lack of resources, short-term contracts, and the sporadic nature of research careers (Iwaniec and McCrystal 1999; Hughes *et al.* 2000). Dissemination is further limited by the fact that 'research activity' within the research community is judged primarily by the number of publications in high-quality research journals (Broad 1999). However, these are not the publications that practitioners tend to read (Iwaniec and Pinkerton 1998; Sheldon and Macdonald 1999; Hughes *et al.* 2000).

Promoting awareness of research evidence is seen as the first step towards its potential use (Anderson *et al.* 1999), and the widespread availability of evidence is clearly of primary importance (Davis and Taylor-Vaisey 1997). However, there is also a need for a detailed implementation strategy (Davis and Taylor-Vaisey 1997). The success of this is largely dependent upon whether research is accessible or not.

Is research evidence accessible?

For us accessibility can be viewed in two main ways. First, practitioners must be able to obtain the evidence, and secondly, having done so, they must be able to understand it.

The infrastructures set up to make research accessible to practitioners are very different in health and social care arenas. Many health service organizations have well-resourced health science libraries, whereas in social care, library facilities and resources vary considerably and depend largely on the investment made within local authorities. Many departments have only a small room with a limited number of books.

Investment in Internet access and developing IT skills within the workforce also varies widely within social care (see for example the audit undertaken by Research in Practice at www.rip.org.uk; accessed 26 June 2002). However, there is some evidence to suggest that even when a good infrastructure is in place, social care practitioners have difficulties in engaging with new technologies (Phillips and Berman 1995).

On the national level, social care is also some way behind health in the use of communication and information technology, for example, the Electronic Library for Social Care (eLSC) has only recently been developed, based on the principles of the National Electronic Library for Health, NELH, and is less well resourced.

However, certain initiatives have been shown to make research more accessible to practitioners, mainly in the field of child care (see, for example, the Children Looked After Materials and Quality Protects initiative at www.doh.gov.uk/qualityprotects/; accessed 26 June 2002). This highlights the potential for increasing access to research using initiatives such as the NSF for older people.

Even when evidence is widely available practitioners often struggle to understand its message. This is due in part to the difficulties of critical appraisal and the relative lack of skill among practitioners (Hughes *et al.* 2000; Smith *et al.* 2001), but the situation is compounded by the status accorded to peer-reviewed sources, which are not necessarily the most accessible, either physically or conceptually. For example, evidence suggests that nearly three-quarters of practitioners do not feel that research is easy to read and understand (Nolan *et al.* 1998).

Clearly, better education and training, together with more user-friendly methods of dissemination, are all important, but these alone are not likely to be sufficient to ensure that the research is adopted into practice (Davis and Taylor-Vaisey 1997; Abbott and Hutchkins 2001). Several other barriers must also be addressed.

Is the research adopted?

The 'messy business' of applying research in practice has been more extensively investigated in health than in social care settings (Hughes *et al.* 2000). Much of the literature strongly points to the need to invest in implementation as well as dissemination strategies. Such implementation strategies should stem from an appreciation of the barriers to implementation that exist (NHS Centre for Reviews and Dissemination 1999), overcoming which may require a series of initiatives such as reminder systems, clinical

Table 15.1   Barriers to using research

	UK[1]	Australia[2]	Sweden[3]	USA[4]
Insufficient time	1	1	5	2
Insufficient resources	2	5	2	8
Nurses' lack of authority to change practice	3	7	6	1
Statistics difficult to understand	4	4	10	9
Research difficult to read/understand	5	12	12	7
Uncooperative doctors	6	6	13	4
Insufficient time to read research	7	2	4	10
Other staff uncooperative	8	8	15	6
Not knowing what evidence is available	9	3	14	3
Evidence is not available in one place	10	19	8	12

[1] *Source*: Nolan *et al.* 1998
[2] *Source*: Retsas and Nolan 1999
[3] *Source*: Kajermo *et al.* 1998
[4] *Source*: Funk *et al.* 1991

audit with feedback, educational outreach (NHS Centre for Reviews and Dissemination 1999), and facilitation in the workplace (Kitson *et al.* 1998).

Abbott and Hutchkins (2001) contend that an essential first step is to ensure that evidence is familiar, comprehensive and credible to practitioners, and that a realistic implementation strategy is adopted, underpinned by an awareness of the potential barriers. Such barriers may be formidable and it is important that there is investment in both individuals and organizations so as to increase their capacity to address existing impediments (Muir-Gray 1997). Muir-Gray (1997) argues that this requires a three-phase strategy which promotes motivation to use research, the competence needed to use research and the ability to overcome barriers. Although such barriers may vary, several studies in nursing have identified a very similar list. Nolan *et al.* (1999) illustrate this by comparing data they collected in the UK and Australia with data obtained from studies using the same instrument in the USA and Sweden. The barriers they identified are summarized in Table 15.1, which lists the top 10 perceived barriers from the UK study and then considers how they relate to the other countries.

Although there is some variation in the above results they also share a great deal in common, with most of the significant barriers relating to the organization itself in terms of insufficient time and resources, but also a perceived lack of authority.

Newman *et al.* (1998) reached a similar conclusion, citing a formidable list of organizational barriers to the use of research including:

- failure to prioritize evidence-based care;
- top-down management approach;

- limited systems for personal and professional development;
- absence of a systematic approach to managing innovation;
- poor communication;
- limited library access;
- resource constraints.

Clearly the creation of an open and flexible organizational culture, with sufficient resources, is essential if research is to be more widely adopted. For example see Box 15.2 below.

Box 15.2   REAL team working

The Research in Practice initiative has started to get the implementation of evidence into practice through the REAL (Reflection, Evidence, Action Learning) team-working project, culminating in the development of an action pack. The pack is the result of several stages of working with teams across different social service departments, combining 'evidence' from working at the coalface of practice in a reflective way, and 'evidence' from research. The pack contains a 'tool kit' which points to mechanisms that seem to work in some contexts including: one-to-one and group supervision of social workers, developing topic work with evaluation at its core, using trigger events such as case reviews to ensure the use of evidence is sought and implemented, and involving service users in planning.

(Barratt and Cooke 2001)

Moving the agenda forward: practitioner and user involvement

Attention to the five As provides one way of improving the current situation, but we would also suggest that other more radical approaches are needed so as to empower practitioners and older people. This will require a range of differing methodologies such as action research (Hart and Bond 2000) and emancipatory approaches (Beresford 1999; Braye 2000); see also Peace in this volume.

The development of the practitioner researcher has been welcomed in both social work and nursing (Shaw 1999), being predicated on models of participatory inquiry where the 'researched' and 'researcher' work together as partners with a commitment to five shared principles (Cancian and Armstead quoted in Shaw 1999):

- the participation of those being studied;
- respect for popular knowledge in agreeing, conducting, and reporting research. This includes the 'tacit' knowledge of practitioners;
- a focus on issues of empowerment;
- an educative dimension through consciousness raising;
- political action and social transformation.

Such an approach fits comfortably with the caring professions where there is a growing emphasis on reflection, which is 'indigenous to practice rather than being on loan from research or evaluation methodology' (Shaw 1999: 115). For example, Shaw and Shaw (1997) report on in-depth interviews conducted with social care practitioners, which illustrated how practitioners adopt a critical approach to their own practice (self-evaluation rather than evaluation with a capital E), explicitly related to professional values, supporting a more 'humanist' approach to social care evaluation based on existing practice skills. They propose engaging and building on these skills to shape a realistic evidence base grounded in practice:

> We need to work 'from the bottom up', grounding our model of evaluation in practitioner's own accounts, rather than superimposing an ideal model 'from the top down' which will necessarily lack meaning in the context of everyday social work practice.
>
> (Shaw and Shaw 1997: 862)

Methods can be diverse and wide-ranging, including in-depth interviewing, life histories, as well as focus groups, case studies, and member validating exercises that contribute to the information used in the cycles of reflection (Shaw and Shaw 1997). Such beliefs clearly resonate with the other contributors to this book.

Emancipatory inquiry methodologies also include cooperative inquiry, action research, action science and participatory action research (Shaw 1999), underpinned by the belief that knowledge and action are linked. Reason writes 'while understanding and action are logically separate, they cannot be separate in life: so a science of persons must be a science of action' (Reason 1994: 10). Hart and Bond (2000) have written extensively about the use of action research in health and social care, and further suggest that research should focus more on issues in their social context. They advocate the exploration of issues from differing (and sometimes divergent) perspectives in order to plan change. Such evidence is potentially more useful to practice because it addresses concerns that have been identified from within the real world.

The last decade has seen considerable emphasis placed on exploring ways in which older people and their carers can be empowered to play a much greater part in the design and delivery of services (Bernard and Phillips 2000). See Peace in this volume for a discussion of this. Despite this it seems that the current inequalities in health experienced by older people may be exacerbated in the future (Minkler 1996; Scheidt *et al.* 1999).

Participatory approaches have direct relevance for working in partnership with service users, and are particularly appropriate to working with marginalized groups such as older adults (Shaw and Shaw 1997; Braye 2000). The consumer movement within the NHS suggests that users can be involved at any stage of the research process including making decisions about what to research, data collection, analysis and dissemination (Hanley *et al.* 2000). However, involvement can mean different things, and can cover the spectrum of power sharing from consultation, through collaboration, to active user control (Hanley *et al.* 2000). Barnes and Wistow (1992) emphasize the importance of applying empowerment theory to user involvement research by adopting a participatory approach where users share research decisions (Elden 1981; Beresford 1992). To date little user-controlled, emancipatory research has been undertaken or funded by the NHS, and most is supported by charitable trusts (Hanley *et al.* 2000), with Warren and Maltby (2000) concluding that involving older people in participatory research is still in its infancy, and assessment of impact is rare. If the situation is to improve it is important to engage in more constructive debate about the value of a more inclusive approach to research. For example, Shaw (2000) outlines five requirements for participatory inquiry. These are to:

- clarify and agree the purpose of participation;
- clarify different kinds of user;
- establish mechanisms for collaboration;
- seek agreement on the risks involved;
- agree 'what's in it for the collaborators', how harm can be avoided and the benefits to be gained by those who collaborate.

Involvement needs to be handled sensitively, especially when working with vulnerable older adults, but participation at any level may be beneficial. Littlechild and Glasby (2000) point out that even very vulnerable adults can contribute meaningfully with adequate support and encouragement.

As Barnes and Warren (1999) contend, 'new voices' from previously silent and disadvantaged groups, including older people, are beginning to exert an influence as teachers and researchers, with groups of service users inputting to the training of practitioners and playing active roles in the research process. However, despite encouraging developments they believe that it is difficult to publish such innovations or to persuade funders of their merit because agendas are still dominated by the concerns of service commissioners and providers.

Conclusion

Warren (1999) argues that genuine improvements will prove elusive until greater prominence is accorded to the needs of frail older people, and those who currently hold the balance of power can overcome their fears of losing their 'expert' status. She contends that exploring some of the above tensions should become increasingly important questions for the research community. This challenge is captured eloquently thus:

> One potentially disempowering aspect of traditional research practice has been the typically exclusive focus of researchers on the technical aspects of process and a failure to consider its 'social' aspects.
>
> (Barnes and Warren 1999: 7)

Although Barnes and Warren are referring to the barriers which limit the involvement of disadvantaged groups, we would argue that these sentiments are just as relevant to the wider issue of 'using' research in gerontology. Essentially more attention to the 'social' nature of research is a prerequisite to making it more 'user-friendly', whether this be in terms of the involvement of stakeholders as researchers, debates as to what constitutes 'evidence', or strategies for dissemination or implementation.

References

Abbott, S. and Hutchkins, J. (2001) It takes more than clinical effectiveness to change nursing practice: an unsuccessful project in the nurse promotion of urinary incontinence, *Clinical Effectiveness in Nursing*, 5(2): 81–7.

Adams, A., Heasman, P. and Gilbert, L. (1999) Opportunities and constraints to practitioner research in the personal social services, *Research, Policy and Planning*, 17: 1.

Anderson, M., Costing, J., Swan, B., Moore, H. and Brookhaven, M. (1999) The use of research in local health agencies, *Social Science and Medicine*, 49: 1007–19.

Barnes, M. and Warren, L. (1999) *Paths to Empowerment*. Bristol: The Policy Press.

Barnes, M. and Wistow, G. (1992) Researcher and user involvement: contributions to learning and methods, in M. Barnes and G. Wistow (eds) *Researching User Involvement*. Leeds: Nuffield Institute of Health.

Barratt, M. and Cooke, J. (2001) *Real Teams Action Pack. Evidence-based Practice in Teams*. Sheffield: Children and Families Unit, University of Sheffield.

Bengston, V.L., Burgess, E.O. and Parrat, T.M. (1997) Theory, explanation and a third generation of theoretical development in social gerontology, *Journal of Gerontology (Social Series)*, 52(2): 572–88.

Beresford, P. (1992) Researching user involvement: a collaborating or colonising enterprise?, in M. Barnes and G. Wistow (eds) *Researching User Involvement*. Leeds: Nuffield Institute of Health.

Beresford, P. (1999) Service users' knowledges and social work theory: conflict or collaboration? At http://www.nisw.org.uk/tswr/beresfordedinburgh.html (accessed 26 June 2002).

Bernard, M. and Phillips, J. (2000) The challenge of ageing in tomorrow's Britain, *Ageing and Society*, 20(1): 33–54.

Black, D. (2001) The limitations of evidence, in T. Heller, R. Muston, M. Siddell and C. Lloyd (eds) *Working for Health*, pp. 28–34. London: Sage Publications.

Braye, S. (2000) Participation and involvement in social care: an overview, in H. Kemshall and R. Littlechild (eds) *User Involvement and Participation in Social Care*. London: Jessica Kingsley.

Brechin, A. and Siddell, M. (2000) Ways of knowing, in R. Gomm and C. Davies (eds) *Using Evidence in Health and Social Care*. London: Sage Publications/The Open University.

Broad, B. (1999) The politics of social work research and evaluation, *Research, Policy and Planning*, 17: 1.

Clarke, J.B. (1999) Evidence-based practice: a retrograde step? The importance of pluralism in evidence generation for the practice of health care, *Journal of Clinical Nursing*, 8(1): 89–94.

Davis, D.A. and Taylor-Vaisey, A. (1997) Translating guidelines into practice: a systematic review of thematic concepts, practical experience and research evidence in the adoption of clinical practice guidelines, *Canadian Medical Association*, 154(4): 408–16.

Department of Health (1996) *Promoting Clinical Effectiveness. A Framework for Action in and through the NHS*. Leeds: Department of Health.

Department of Health (2001) *Research Governence Framework for Health and Social Care*. London: Department of Health.

Dunn, V., Chricton, N., Williams, K., Roe, B. and Sears, K. (1998) Using research for practice: a UK experience of the BARRIERS scale, *Journal of Advanced Nursing*, 1203–10.

Elden, M. (1981) Sharing the research work: participative research and its role demands, in P. Reason and J. Rowan (eds) *Human Inquiry*. Chichester: John Wiley.

Fisher, M. (2000) A Strategic Framework for Social Work Research. At http://www.nisw.org.uk/tswr/strategicframework.html (accessed 26 June 2002).

Funk, S.G., Champagne, M.T., Wiese, R.A. and Tornquist, E.M. (1991) BARRIERS: The barriers to research utilisation scale, *Applied Nursing Research*, 4: 39–45.

Gomm, R. (2000) Evidence for planning services, in R. Gomm and C. Davies (eds) *Using Evidence in Health and Social Care*. London: Sage Publications/The Open University.

Hanley, B., Bradburn, J., Gorin, S. *et al.* (2000) *Involving Consumers in Research and Development in the NHS: Briefing Notes for Researchers*. Winchester: Help for Health Trust.

Hart, E. and Bond, M. (2000) Using action research, in R. Gomm and C. Davies (eds) *Using Evidence in Health and Social Care*. London: Sage Publications/The Open University.

Hughes, M., McNeish, D., Newman, T., Roberts, H. and Sachdev, D. (2000) *Making Connections: Linking Research and Practice*. Essex: Barnardo's.

Hunt, J. (1981) Indication for nursing practice: the use of research findings, *Journal of Advanced Nursing*, 61: 189–94.

Hunt, J. (1996) Barriers to research utilization, *Journal of Advanced Nursing*, 23: 423–5.

Iwaniec, D. and McCrystal, P. (1999) The centre for childcare research at Queen's University, Belfast, *Research on Social Work and Practice*, 9: 248–60.

Iwaniec, D. and Pinkerton, J. (1998) *Making Research Work: Promoting Child Care Policy and Practice*. Chichester: Wiley.

James, T. and Smith, P. (1999) Implementing research: the practice, in A. Mullall and A. Le May (eds) *Nursing Research: Dissemination and Implementation*, pp. 177–204. Edinburgh: Churchill Livingstone.

Kajermo, K.N., Nordstrom, G., Krusebrant, A. and Bjorvell, H. (1998) Barriers to and facilitation of research utilization as perceived by a group of registered nurses in Sweden, *Journal of Advanced Nursing*, 27: 798–807.

Kitson, A., Harvey, G. and McCormack, B. (1998) Enabling the implementation of evidence based practice: a conceptual framework, *Quality in Health*, 7: 149–58.

Le May, A. (1999) Evidence-based practice, *Nursing Times*, Monograph No. 1. London: *Nursing Times*.

Littlechild, R. and Glasby, J. (2000) Older people as participating patients, in H. Kemshall and R. Littlechild (eds) *User Involvement and Participation in Social Care*. London: Jessica Kingsley.

McCrystal, P. (2000) Developing the social work researcher through a practitioner research training programme, *Social Work Education*, 19(4): 359–73.

McSherry, R. (1997) What do registered nurses know and feel about research?, *Journal of Advanced Nursing*, 25(5): 985–98.

Minkler, M. (1996) Critical perspectives on ageing: new challenges for gerontology, *Ageing and Society*, 16(4): 467–87.

Muir-Gray, J.A. (1997) *Evidence-based Health Care. How To Make Health Policy and Management Decisions*. Edinburgh: Churchill Livingstone.

Needham, G. (2000) Research and practice: making a difference, in R. Gomm and C. Dawes (eds) *Using Evidence in Health and Social Care*, pp. 131–51. London: Sage Publications.

Newman, M., Papadopoulos, I. and Sigsworth, J. (1998) Barriers to evidence-based practice, *Clinical Effectiveness in Nursing*, 2(1): 11–20.

NHS Centre for Reviews and Dissemination (1999) Getting evidence into practice, *Effective Health Care*, 5(1): 1–16.

Nolan, M.R., Morgan, L., Curran, M. *et al.* (1998) Evidence-based care: can we overcome the barriers? *British Journal of Nursing*, 7: 1273–8.

Nolan, M.R., Marsh, G. and Retsas, A. (1999) Implementing evidence-based care: overcoming the barriers. Paper presented at ICN Congress, London, June.

Osborn, A. and Willcocks, D. (1990) Making Research Useful and Usable, in S.M. Peace (ed.) *Researching Social Gerontology: Concepts, Methods and Issues*. London: Sage Publications.

Pearlin, L.I., Harrington, C., Powell-Lawton, M., Montgomery, R.J.V. and Zarit, S.H. (2001) An overview of the social and behavioural consequences of Alzheimer's disease, *Aging and Mental Health*, 5(Supplement 1): S3–S6.

Phillips, D. and Berman, Y. (1995) *Human Services in the Age of New Technology: Harmonising Social Work and Computerisation*. Aldershot: Avebury.

Reason, P. (1994) Inquiry and alienation, in P. Reason (ed.) *Participation in Human Inquiry*. London: Sage Publications.

Retsas, A.P. and Nolan, M.R. (1999) Barriers to nurses' use of research: an Australian hospital study, *International Journal of Nursing Studies*, 36: 335–43.

Rossi, P. and Freeman, H.E. (1993) *Evaluation: A Systematic Approach*, 5th edition. Newbury Park: Sage Publications.

Sackett, D., Rosenberg, W. and Muir-Gray, J.A. (1996) Evidence-based medicine: what it is and what it isn't, *British Medical Journal*, 312: 71–2.

Scheidt, R.J., Humphreys, D.R. and Yorgason, J.B. (1999) Successful ageing: what's not to like?, *Journal of Applied Gerontology*, 18(8): 277–82.

Shaw, I. (1999) *Qualitative Evaluation*. London: Sage Publications.

Shaw, I. (2000) Just inquiry? Research and evaluation for service users, in H. Kemshall and R. Littlechild (eds) *User Involvement and Participation in Social Care*. London: Jessica Kingsley.

Shaw, I. and Shaw, A. (1997) Keeping social work honest: evaluating as profession and practice, *British Journal of Social Work*, 27: 847–69.

Sheldon, B. and Macdonald, G. (1999) *Research and Practice in Social Care: Mind the Gap*. Exeter: Centre for Evidence-based Social Services.

Smith, D. (2000) What works as evidence for practice? The methodological repertoire in an applied discipline at http://www.nisw.org.uk/tswr/smith.html (accessed 26 June 2002).

Smith, H., Owen, J., Marsh, P. and Cooke, J. (2001) *Developing Research at the Social Services and Health Interface*. Sheffield: University of Sheffield.

Walsh, M.P. (1998) What is evidence? A critical view for nursing, *Journal of Clinical Effectiveness*, 2(2): 86–93.

Warren, L. (1999) Empowerment: the path to partnership, in M. Barnes and L. Warren (eds) *Paths to Empowerment*. Bristol: The Policy Press.

Warren, L. and Maltby, T. (2000) Involving older people in change, in T. Warnes, L. Warren and M. Nolan (eds) *Care Services for Later Life: Transformations and Critiques*. London: Jessica Kingsley.

Web resources*

1 Professional associations in gerontology

British Society of Gerontology – http://www.soc.surrey.ac.uk/bsg/
The Gerontological Society of America – http://www.geron.org/
The International Association of Gerontology – http://www.sfu.ca/iag/

2 Organizations relating to policy and practice

Age Concern England – http://www.ace.org.uk/
Links to a wide range of organizations and projects for older people.
British Association for Service to the Elderly – http://www.base.org.uk/
Centre for Policy on Ageing – http://www.cpa.org.uk/

3 Research funding sources

Association of Medical Research Charities – http://www.amrc.org.uk/grantsearch/
ukonly.html
Provides information on a variety of medical associations offering research
funding.

* All web sites listed here were last accessed 26 June 2002.

Department of Health – http://www.doh.gov.uk/research/index.htm
Health and social care policy and practice-related research.
Economic and Social Research Council – http://www.esrc.ac.uk/fundops.htm
Lifecourse, Lifestyles and Health.
Social Stability and Exclusion.
Joseph Rowntree Foundation – http://www.jrf.org.uk/funding/default.htm
Housing and Neighbourhood priorities (HANC).
Social Care and Disability priorities (SCDC).
Work, Income and Social Policy priorities (WISP).
The Nuffield Foundation – http://www.nuffieldfoundation.org/award/
  index.html
Social Science.
Science (Research Grants, Education, Rheumatism and Arthritis Research).
Ageing.
Regional Health Authorities each have their own websites
For example, for West Midlands – http://www.doh.gov.uk/research/wmro/
  funding.htm
Refund List – http://www.refund.ncl.ac.uk/RefundNew/Site/grantfunders.htm
Research funding information service covering many different areas of
  research.
The Wellcome Trust – http://www.wellcome.ac.uk/
Medicine and Disease.

4 Statistical sources, data sets and research information

ALSPAC – http://www.ich.bris.ac.uk/alspac.html
Information about the Avon Longitudinal Study of Parents and Children,
  ALSPAC study.
The Census site – http://www.census.ac.uk
Centre for Longitudinal Studies, Institute of Education – http://www.cls.ioe.ac.uk
Information about the 1958 study, the National Child Development Study
  (also known as the 1958 British Birth Cohort Study), the 1970 British
  Birth Cohort Study, and the Millennium Birth Cohort Study.
http://www.iser.essex.ac.uk/bhps/-
Data and information about the British Household Panel Survey.
Department of Health – http://www.doh.gov.uk-
Many full text publications available; data in the statistics and surveys
  section covers all aspects of the health service including waiting times,
  hospital utilization and summaries of research reports.
The ESRC Growing Older Programme – http://www.shef.ac.uk/uni/project/gop
Information about projects involved in the ESRC funded research
  programme.
The Medical Research Council – http://www.mrc.ac.uk

Information about the MRC National Survey of Health and Development.
Office for National Statistics – http://www.statistics.gov.uk
Contains many full text ONS publications, data sets and student resources.
Comprehensive guide to government survey and statistical data and many
  data sets can be downloaded directly.
UK data archive site – http://www.data-archive.ac.uk-
Comprehensive list of data and links to international data sets.
United Nations – http://www.un.org
For global statistics.
University of Essex archive of qualitative data – http://www.essex.ac.uk/qualidata
World Health Organization – http://www.who.int-
International health data, and on:
http://www.who.int/m/healthtopics-a-z/en/index.html-
A–Z of health topics.

5 Specialist photographic and related collections

The Centre for the Study of Cartoons and Caricature, University of Kent – http://
  library.ukc.ac.uk/cartoons
National Museum of Photography, Film and Television – http://www.nmpft.org.uk/
  research/information.asp
National Museums of Scotland. Museum of Scottish Country Life – http://
  www.nms.ac.uk/agriculture/
North Highland Archive – http://www.caithness.org/community/museums/
  nha/indexes/plist.htm
Shetland Museums Service – http://www.scottish-fisheries-museum.org/
St Andrews University Library Special Collections – http://ibasenet.st-and.ac.uk
The Sutcliffe Gallery – http://www.sutcliffe-gallery.co.uk

6 The Mass Observation Archive

The Mass Observation Archive – http://www.sussex.ac.uk/library/massobs
The MOA *Database of contributors* – http://www.sussex.ac.uk/library/massobs/
  diaries_and_personal_writing_1937–65.html

7 Sources on race, ethnicity and ageing

Ageing and Ethnicity Web – http://www.aeweb.org/index.html
Centre for Research in Ethnic Relations, Warwick University – http://www.
  warwick.ac.uk/fac/soc/CRER_RC/
The Commission for Racial Equality – http://www.cre.gov.uk/
Crosspoint Anti Racism UK – http://www.magenta.nl/crosspoint/uk.html

Links to anti-racist groups in UK.

Institute of Race Relations – http://www.irr.org.uk

Race Equality in the Department of Health – http://www.doh.gov.uk/race_
equality/climate.htm

Reminiscence Theatre for Minority Older People – http://www.aeweb.org/
methods/reminiscence.htm

8 Research ethics guidelines

British Psychological Society Code of Practice – http://www.bps.org.uk/about/
rules5.cfm/code

British Sociological Association ethics guidelines – http://www.britsoc.org.uk

Medical Research Council on ethics – http://www.mrc.ac.uk/index/publications/
publications_ethics_and_best_practice.htm

Oral History Society – http://www.oralhistory.org.uk

Information about 'Copyright and ethics'.

Social Research Association – http://www.the-sra.org.uk/index2.htm

Index

Page numbers in *italics* refer to tables, figures and boxes.